# REDUCING THE RISK

## *BUILDING SKILLS TO PREVENT*

# PREGNANCY STD & HIV

THIRD EDITION

RICHARD P. BARTH, MSW, PHD

FOREWORD BY DOUGLAS KIRBY, PHD

ETR ASSOCIATES
Santa Cruz, California
1996

ETR Associates (Education, Training and Research) is a nonprofit organization committed to fostering the health, well-being and cultural diversity of individuals, families, schools and communities. The publishing program of ETR Associates provides books and materials that empower young people and adults with the skills to make positive health choices. We invite health professionals to learn more about our high-quality resources and our training and research programs by contacting us at P.O. Box 1830, Santa Cruz, CA 95061-1830.

 Published by ETR Associates, P.O. Box 1830, Santa Cruz, CA 95061-1830, 1-800-321-4407.
Printed in the United States of America

10 9 8 7 6

Cover design: Cliff Warner

Title No. 359

**Library of Congress Cataloging-in-Publication Data**

Barth, Richard P., 1952–
Reducing the risk : building skills to prevent pregnancy, STD & HIV / Richard P. Barth. —3rd ed.
p. cm.
Includes bibliographical references.
ISBN 1-56071-398-4
1. Sex instruction—United States—Curricula. 2. Birth control—Study and teaching (Secondary)—United States. 3. Sexual abstinence—Study and teaching (Secondary)—United States. I. Title.
HQ57.5.A3B27 1995
613.9'071'2—dc20 95-30962

*The development of this curriculum was made possible by grants from the Stuart Foundations and the U.S. Centers for Disease Control. The opinions expressed are those of the author and do not necessarily reflect those of the Stuart Foundations and the U.S. Centers for Disease Control.*

# CONTENTS

# PUBLISHER'S NOTE

## Program Intent

The major focus of *Reducing the Risk: Building Skills to Prevent Pregnancy, STD and HIV* is the practice of communication skills to prevent pregnancy and the transmission of STD. A primary goal of prevention efforts with teens is to educate them to change risk behaviors and to practice behaviors that eliminate or reduce the risk of pregnancy or STD, including HIV infection.

*Reducing the Risk* was developed with the specific intent of influencing adolescent sexual and drug behaviors. This curriculum is designed to be embedded in the context of a comprehensive family life or health education program and is particularly appropriate in communities where there are high rates of teen pregnancy, drug use and sexually transmitted disease.

Some of the material is controversial due to the nature of the subject matter covered. The laws relating to teaching sensitive topics in the classroom vary throughout the country and will have an effect on what may be taught and how it is presented. We recommend that teachers understand and apply district policies and state mandates and obtain parent, school board and administrative support before using the material. We also encourage teachers to adapt the dialogue of the role plays to make them more culturally and/or regionally appropriate.

## New to the Third Edition

*Reducing the Risk* was originally published in 1989. The second edition, published in 1993, expanded on the first by augmenting the material on HIV prevention. The third edition has been further revised and/or updated in the following ways:

- Information about birth control and sexually transmitted disease, including HIV, was reviewed and revisions made based on the most current research about protection and prevention.
- The instructional process for teaching refusals and delaying tactics were enhanced based on the extensive experience of ETR Associates' training staff, who have worked with thousands of teachers in implementing the program.

- Information to help in the implementation of *Reducing the Risk* has been added as appendixes. These include: (1) most frequently asked questions and answers about the curriculum, (2) how to use role plays, and (3) answering student questions.
- A Spanish-language student workbook is now available.
- An optional supplementary kit of materials, including skill posters and role play cards, is available.

# FOREWORD

Since the mid-1970s when this country's concern about teenage pregnancy became heightened, there has been a search for sexuality education programs to reduce behaviors that place youth at risk of pregnancy. Since the mid-1980s when concern about AIDS and HIV became heightened, there has also been a search for HIV education programs that reduce behaviors which may transmit HIV and other STDs.

Hundreds of sexuality education and HIV education curricula have been developed and implemented in junior and senior high schools during the last 15 years. Unfortunately, most of these curricula have not been evaluated, or, when they have been evaluated, the results have indicated that the curricula did not significantly reduce unprotected intercourse.

Because of the importance of identifying and replicating effective programs, the Centers for Disease Control and Prevention periodically reviews all research studies on school-based curricula designed to reduce unprotected sexual intercourse, either by delaying intercourse or increasing condom and contraceptive use. As this foreword is being written, there are only three curricula that the Centers for Disease Control and Prevention has found to have been well evaluated and to have significantly reduced unprotected intercourse. *Reducing the Risk* is one of those three.

The *Reducing the Risk (RTR)* curriculum is one of the first rigorously evaluated sexuality education curricula to have a measurable impact upon behavior (Kirby, Barth, Leland and Fetro, 1991). It was the first to be evaluated in a high school setting and to have employed such methodological advances as large sample sizes, good comparison/control groups and long-term follow-up. In 13 high schools throughout California, 46 classrooms were assigned to program and comparison groups. Questionnaires measuring knowledge, peer norms, behavioral intentions, sexual and contraceptive behaviors and parent/child communication were administered to these students before the curriculum was implemented, immediately after the curriculum was implemented, about six months later and about 18 months later. A total of 758 students were tracked for 18 months. Results indicated that, among all youth, the curriculum significantly increased knowledge and that students retained this greater knowledge for at least 18 months.

One of the goals of this norm- and skills-based curriculum was to change norms about unprotected sex and to change students' perceptions that "everyone is doing it." The *RTR* curriculum apparently did not diminish the perceived proportions of students their age who had ever had sex, but did apparently prevent those perceptions from becoming worse over time.

The curriculum increased parent/child communication about abstinence and contraception. According to both students and parents, the curriculum also made this communication easier. About one-fourth of the sampled parents indicated that this was the first time they had discussed these topics with their children.

Among students who had not initiated intercourse prior to the pretest, the curriculum significantly reduced the onset of intercourse at 18 months—the proportional reduction was 24 percent. Among those relatively few students who did initiate intercourse after the curriculum was implemented, larger percentages of the program group than of the comparison group used contraceptives. Thus, an analysis of measures of unprotected intercourse (derived from both abstinence and use of contraceptives) revealed that the curriculum significantly reduced unprotected intercourse among all students who had not initiated intercourse at pretest. These effects extended across a variety of sub-groups, including at least two different ethnic groups, both sexes, and lower- and higher-risk youth, but the curriculum was particularly effective for lower-risk youth and female students.

About one-third (37 percent) of the sample had initiated intercourse prior to the program. In part because of the smaller sample size, it was more difficult to determine the impact of *RTR* upon contraceptive use in this sample. For this entire sample of youth who had initiated intercourse prior to the program, there were no statistically significant differences in the increase in contraceptive use between the *RTR* group and the control group. On some measures, the *RTR* group did report greater increases in contraceptive use than did the comparison group, but these increases were not statistically significant. However, among females and among lower-risk youth who had initiated intercourse prior to the program, the *RTR* group had statistically significantly greater increases in contraceptive use than did the comparison group.

Overall, these results are particularly impressive given that most of the students in the comparison groups received a more traditional sexuality education course of the same length. Thus, these data suggest that *Reducing the Risk* is more effective at producing these desired behavioral changes than are more traditional curricula.

A review of curricula that effectively change sexual risk-taking behavior, as well as curricula that did not change behavior, indicates that the effective curricula share the following eight characteristics, which may be linked to their success, while the ineffective curricula lack one or more of these characteristics (Kirby, 1995).

1. Effective programs included a narrow focus on reducing sexual risk-taking behaviors that may lead to HIV/STD infection or unintended pregnancy. The *Reducing the Risk* curriculum does this by focusing upon delaying the onset of intercourse and using protection if intercourse occurs.
2. In general, the effective programs were based upon theoretical approaches that have been demonstrated to be effective in influencing other health risk behaviors, e.g., social cognitive theory, social influence theory, social inoculation theory, cognitive behavioral theory, and the theory of reasoned action. *Reducing the Risk* is based upon social cognitive theory, social influence theory and social inoculation theory.
3. Effective programs tended to fall into two categories, those that lasted 14 or more hours, and those that lasted a smaller number of hours but implemented the curriculum in small group settings with a leader for each group and could therefore

use the limited time more effectively. Longer programs provided the opportunity to complete many of the activities discussed below. *Reducing the Risk* lasts 16 hours.

4. Effective programs employed a variety of teaching methods designed to involve the participants and have them personalize the information. Instructors reached students through active learning methods rather than didactic instruction. In *Reducing the Risk* students are involved in numerous experiential classroom and homework activities: small group discussions; games or simulations; brainstorming; role playing with written rehearsal, practice, verbal feedback and coaching; locating contraception in local drugstores; visiting or telephoning family planning clinics; and interviewing parents.

5. Effective programs provided basic information that students needed to assess risks and avoid unprotected sex. Typically, this information was not unnecessarily detailed or comprehensive. Instead, the programs emphasized the basic facts needed to make behaviorally relevant decisions. *Reducing the Risk* provides this type of information.

6. Effective programs included activities that addressed social pressures on sexual behaviors. *Reducing the Risk* does this in several ways. It discusses situations that might lead to sex, discusses "lines" typically used to get someone to have sex, and provides role playing situations to help students respond to these "lines" and avoid potentially risky situations.

7. Effective programs reinforced clear and appropriate values in order to strengthen individual values and group norms against unprotected sex (i.e., postponing sex, avoiding unprotected intercourse, using condoms, and avoiding high-risk partners). The values and norms expressed in these programs were tailored for the age and experience of the target population. The *Reducing the Risk* curriculum conveys the message that students should avoid unprotected intercourse, that abstinence is the best way to do this, and that, if students have sex, they should use protection.

8. Effective programs provided modeling and practice of communication and negotiation skills. *Reducing the Risk* provides information about these skills, models effective use of the skills, and then provides skill rehearsal and practice (e.g., role playing or written practice).

In addition to these eight characteristics of effective curricula, effective programs also provided training for the educators implementing the program. This training ranged from approximately six hours to three days. In general, the training was designed to give teachers and peers information on the program as well as practice in using the teaching strategies included in the curriculum (e.g., conducting role plays and leading group discussions).

The *Reducing the Risk* curriculum is not a total solution to the problems of unprotected intercourse. Unfortunately, there are no "magic bullets" that completely eliminate unprotected intercourse among adolescents. However, this curriculum, when implemented by well-trained teachers, can be an effective component of a more comprehensive program.

Douglas Kirby, PhD
Research Director, ETR Associates

**References**

Kirby, D., R. Barth, N. Leland and J. V. Fetro. 1991. Reducing the risk: Impact of a new curriculum on sexual risk-taking. *Family Planning Perspectives* 23 (6): 253-263.

Kirby, D. 1995. A review of educational programs designed to reduce sexual risk-taking behaviors among school-aged youth in the United States. Washington, DC: U.S. Congress, Office of Technology Assessment.

# PREFACE AND ACKNOWLEDGMENTS

The risks of unprotected sexual intercourse grow greater every day for adolescents. The great personal upheaval that adolescent pregnancy causes is dwarfed by the implications of becoming HIV-infected. Adolescents are among the groups with the greatest growth in the risk of becoming HIV-infected. About 20 percent of all diagnosed AIDS cases in the United States are people between the ages of 20 and 29.

Young people usually want to avoid pregnancy and HIV infection. The ways to do this are to abstain from sex or to use condoms and foam **consistently** and **effectively**. Many youth will be most comfortable abstaining from sex—this curriculum teaches them what they need to know and do to abstain. Other youth will risk pregnancy and HIV unless they protect themselves. To abstain or protect themselves, teens must not only know the risk of pregnancy and HIV but what to do to abstain or protect themselves and how to manage social situations so that they can.

The need for an effective program to delay sexual activity and prevent pregnancy and HIV infection has never been greater. Nearly 70 percent of high school students report that they have had sexual intercourse (Centers for Disease Control and Prevention, 1994). In addition, more than 40 percent of young women in the United States become pregnant before they reach 20 years of age. About 12 percent of 15- to 19-year-old females—more than a million such teenagers—become pregnant each year, producing one of the highest teenage pregnancy rates of any western industrialized country (Alan Guttmacher Institute, 1994).

Parents increasingly appreciate the need for schools to teach their children ways to prevent pregnancy and sexually transmitted disease, including HIV. National opinion polls consistently show that about 85 percent of parents and other adults favor sexuality education in the schools (Scales and Roper, 1994). In 1992, 70 percent supported condom distribution in schools (Elam, Rose and Gallup, 1992). (The percentage of adults who would support providing abstinence and birth control information, as this curriculum does, is certain to be far higher.) Of course, these parents and many more also want their children to know that abstinence is the only completely safe form of pregnancy and HIV prevention and to know what to do to avoid sex.

The author recognizes that HIV infection and pregnancies are not prevented only by increasing adolescents' knowledge and skill in avoiding or effectively handling peer situations that might otherwise involve unprotected sex. Serious prevention efforts are comprehensive and include increasing opportunities for communication between student and parent and students and school personnel. They involve enhanced health care, extracurricular activities, and jobs and careers that present compelling alternatives to risk taking and early parenthood. Whereas this curriculum is a good complement to such school, church and community activities, it is certainly not a substitute for them.

Many youth engage in risky sexual behavior because they do not know how to prevent pregnancy, they do not anticipate the need for birth control because they don't expect to have sex, or they don't have the skill to use protection. This curriculum hits both of these reasons head on. Much time is spent clarifying what one needs to know to prevent pregnancy and HIV infection and how to identify the signs that a sexual encounter might occur. Youth who complete this curriculum should be neither ignorant about nor surprised by sex. They're not likely to get pregnant or become HIV-infected because they have never had practice telling someone they do not want sex. They won't have sex because it is easier to do than to talk about.

The educational basis for *Reducing the Risk: Building Skills to Prevent Pregnancy, STD and HIV* asserts that learning follows from action. This curriculum requires active student participation in role-play situations that simulate those they are likely to confront outside the classroom. Students will be better prepared for such encounters after practice and rehearsal with difficult situations. Homework provides students the opportunity to interview their parents or guardians about their attitudes regarding abstinence and sexuality, visit stores or clinics that sell or provide condoms and other protection, and anticipate situations that might lead to pregnancy or HIV infection. Through the activities in this curriculum, students obtain information and practice with interpersonal skills to keep from becoming pregnant or HIV-infected. Less active approaches to sexuality education have had little success in reducing unplanned adolescent pregnancies (Stout and Rivara 1989). This approach follows a more promising model that combines cognitive and social skill training (Barth 1986; Barth, Middleton and Wagman 1989; Gilchrist and Schinke 1983). The evidence about the effectiveness of this approach for preventing pregnancy is reviewed in Doug Kirby's foreword and argues for its continued use and development.

The Third Edition of *Reducing the Risk* focuses on updating information about HIV. Additionally, the steps for teaching refusals and delaying tactics were tightened based on the field experience of ETR Associates' training staff, specifically Hector Campos and Julie Taylor. Doug Kirby provided a new foreword that describes the research. These people, along with the Publishing Division staff of ETR Associates, made it possible to provide a timely release for this edition. Their efforts are greatly appreciated.

Parts of this manual are adapted from ETR Associates' excellent sexuality and health education curricula, including *Sex Education: Teacher's Guide and Resource Manual* (Bignell, 1982), *Saying No to Alcohol* (Abbey and Wagman, 1987), and *Teaching AIDS* (Quackenbush and Sargent, 1988). The development was primarily funded by a grant from the Stuart Foundations.

I want to acknowledge the contributions to this curriculum of Michelle Barrett, Kay Clark, Rebecca Dominy, Don Eggleston, Lew Gilchrist, Sharon Ikami, Hene Kelly, Sarah Lamb, Nancy Leland, Susan Marsh, Norma Riccobuono, Jane Robles, John Rodriguez, Evelyn Schwall and Lance Sprague. Ellen Wagman kept this idea alive until it could be tried in the way it deserves. Sandy Ludlow's commitment to this project held up under severe tests. Their ideas, time, suggestions and support were often and graciously given and I hope their faith and courage are rewarded. Nancy Abbey, Kathleen Middleton and Mary Nelson devoted untold hours of their awesome talent to the developing, pilot testing and revising of this curriculum. Without them it would be twice as long and half as useful. They have my lasting gratitude. Nancy Leland, Joyce Fetro and Kevin Volkan observed classes hither and yon and provided invaluable commentary. The pilot teachers also provided astute observations and suggestions despite their hectic schedules. I am especially grateful to the Stuart Foundations for support of this project, and to Ted Lobman for his enthusiasm and ideas. His vision and energy are inspiring and sustaining.

Careful research on this curriculum contributes to our confidence in its appeal and usefulness. Claire Brindis, Joyce Fetro, Lew Gilchrist, Doug Kirby, Nancy Leland and Kevin Volkan have made the kind of creative and informed contributions to the evaluation that are every practitioner-scientist-author's dream. The evaluation of the curriculum's impact also received critical support from the William and Flora Hewlett Foundation and Grant S07-RR07006-22 awarded by the Bio-Medical Research Support Grant Program Division of the National Institute of Health.

An Advisory Committee of school administrators, school board members, teachers and parents offered valuable suggestions and assistance in the writing of the first edition of this curriculum. These talented professionals are listed below.

# ADVISORY COMMITTEE MEMBERS

Ms. Barbara Bissell
Nursing Services
San Mateo County Office of Education
Redwood City, California

Ms. Pat Carson
Parent Education Commission
California Parent Teachers Association
Quincy, California

Ms. Elvira Dundy
Principal
Wilson High School
San Francisco Unified School District
San Francisco, California

Rev. Marilyn Erickson
Associate Director
Planned Parenthood Affiliates of California
Sacramento, California

Ms. Pat Hillman
School Board Member
Tulare Unified School District
Visalia, California

Ms. Gloria Joe
Teacher
Abraham Lincoln High School
San Francisco Unified School District
San Francisco, California

Ms. Margaret Philipps
Vice President - Parent Education
California Parent Teachers Association
Walnut Creek, California

Ms. Jacqui Smith
Nutritional Education Specialist
California Department of Education
Sacramento, California

Ms. Gay Veeh
Teacher
Capistrano Unified School District
San Juan Capistrano, California

Ms. Yvonne Willis-Ash
Teacher
Castlemont Senior High School
Oakland Unified School District
Oakland, California

Dr. Claire Brindis
Institute of Health Policy Studies
University of California
San Francisco, California

Ms. Janice Cobb
Teacher
Roosevelt High School
Fresno Unified School District
Fresno, California

Ms. Alice Encinas
Teacher
Roosevelt High School
Fresno Unified School District
Fresno, California

Mr. Ken Forlow
Principal
La Paloma High School
Liberty Union High School District
Brentwood, California

Dr. Pat Ibanez
Teacher
Capistrano Unified School District
San Juan Capistrano, California

Mr. Jim Johnson
Superintendent
Anderson Valley Unified School District
Boonville, California

Ms. Maria Reza
Coordinator
School Based Health Clinics
Los Angeles Unified School District
Los Angeles, California

Ms. Susan Varner
Consultant
Family Health Services
Sacramento, California

Ms. Beverly White
Program Officer
S.H. Cowell Foundation
San Francisco, California

***While the author seriously considered all input from this group, involvement in the Advisory Committee does not necessarily constitute an endorsement of the curriculum. The author is solely responsible for its content.***

# INTRODUCTION

*Reducing the Risk: Building Skills to Prevent Pregnancy, STD and HIV* goes beyond the facts about abstinence and protection. It presents a powerful, active approach to prevention of teenage pregnancy and protection against HIV and other STD that motivates students to change their high-risk behaviors.

Throughout its 16 well-defined lessons, *Reducing the Risk* clearly emphasizes teaching refusals, delaying tactics and alternative actions students can use to abstain or use protection. Specific guidelines for class activities, background information for teachers, and complete lecture notes are included.

## Major Concepts

Three major program concepts provide the foundation for this curriculum:

1. Abstaining from sexual activity *or* refusing unprotected sexual intercourse are the only responsible alternatives for teenagers.
2. Correct information about pregnancy, protection, and sexually transmitted disease (STD), including transmission of the human immunodeficiency virus (HIV), is essential for responsible sexual behavior.
3. Effective communication skills about abstinence and refusal skills related to unprotected sexual intercourse contribute to responsible sexual behavior.

## Program Objectives

As a result of participating in classes that use this curriculum, students will be able to:

1. Evaluate the risks and lasting consequences of becoming an adolescent parent or becoming infected with HIV or another STD.
2. Recognize that abstaining from sexual activity or using contraception are the only ways to avoid pregnancy, HIV infection and other STD.
3. Conclude that factual information about conception and protection is essential for avoiding teenage pregnancy, HIV infection and other STD.

4. Demonstrate effective communication skills for remaining abstinent and for avoiding unprotected sexual intercourse.

## Information

Although information alone does not keep young people from having sex, becoming infected with HIV or getting pregnant, accurate information about the consequences of unprotected sex may strengthen a youth's resolve not to have sex or not to have it without protection. Knowing that many of their peers do not have sex also helps youth understand they have the option to abstain.

In order for information to influence decisions, students must understand that the information is about them. Students complete several activities that bring the implications of becoming a teenage parent or becoming infected with HIV down to their daily lives. Students also describe their own reasons for abstaining from sex or using protection. They discuss these reasons with parents or guardians and they practice stating their opinion during role plays, class activities and discussions, and homework assignments.

## Social Skills

The greatest emphasis of *Reducing the Risk* is teaching students the interpersonal or social skills they can use to abstain or protect. No judgment is made about which of these responses is best. Rather, students learn that they must consult with their parent(s) and their consciences to decide what to do. The curriculum provides ideas, skills and practice to do it effectively. The key skills are:

**Refusals**—responses that clearly say no in a manner that doesn't jeopardize a good relationship but which leaves no ambiguity about the intent not to have sex or unprotected sex.

**Delaying tactics and alternative actions**—ways to avoid a situation or delay acting until the person has time to decide what to do or say or until she or he is more prepared to implement a decision. These are incompatible with impulsive and unprotected sex.

All skills are first explained and demonstrated by the teacher and then practiced by the students in role plays.

## How the Curriculum Was Developed

The curriculum does not assume that youth have sex primarily because someone else pressures them into it by intimidation or suggesting they will be considered inadequate if they abstain. Our interviews and focus groups with young people quickly countered this simple notion. The pressures to try sex are internal as well as external and stem from pervasive familial and social messages that it is good to try new things, to be curious about the world, and to pursue meaningful loving relationships. This curriculum recognizes the value of these desires but helps students learn skills to prevent such influences from leading to pregnancy or STD infection or both.

The curriculum has four major influences. The first is the adolescent pregnancy social skills training strategies developed by Lewayne Gilchrist, Steven Paul Schinke and their colleagues (whom the author counts himself lucky to be among) in the early 1980s. References to their creative and seminal work are listed at the end of the book. The curriculum also draws on the author's more recent work on social and cognitive skills training (Barth 1986) and coping with adolescent relationships (Barth, Schinke and Maxwell 1985) and high school family life education programs (Barth and Derezotes 1990). Finally, ETR Associates' experience with developing curricula for sexuality education has clarified many elements of a successful curriculum.

Reactions from teenagers have been critical to testing the assumptions and specifics of the curriculum. First, four multi-racial focus groups of tenth graders in urban, suburban and rural communities were questioned about ways to make the exercises more fitting and effective. These groups also generated ideas for new activities. Information gleaned from these teen consultants is incorporated into all aspects of the curriculum: the vignettes, role plays, classroom activities and homework assignments.

The first version of the curriculum was then pilot tested by a total of six ETR Associates staff and teachers in five diverse schools. The settings included two continuation (alternative education) school classes, an English as a Second Language class, and classes in suburban, rural and inner city schools. Every class was observed in at least three different schools. Extensive revisions were completed following this pilot-testing. The revised curriculum was then implemented in 19 classrooms situated in 13 school districts spread across California from a few miles south of Oregon to the edge of the Mexican border. Few, if any, programs to prevent pregnancy have undergone such meticulous development. The seriousness of this topic deserves no less.

## How to Use This Curriculum

Each class includes a synopsis of activities and the approximate time required for each activity, materials needed, detailed steps for leading each activity, student worksheets and handouts, role play scripts, teacher references and homework assignments. There are two options for Class 1: "Class 1" focuses on pregnancy prevention; "Alternate Class 1" focuses on prevention of HIV infection.

The classes are designed for 45-minute periods; however, most can be expanded to fill two periods by increasing practice time and providing more time for discussion and disclosure. Students may initially be hesitant about the expectations for role play performance, but they soon begin to enjoy those opportunities and use them to great advantage. Productive use of the curriculum insists that teachers continue to encourage students to practice their interpersonal skills in role plays. As an old saying goes, "You are what you pretend to be." The more students pretend to effectively say no to sex or to plan to use protection, the more likely it is that they will act that way outside the classroom.

## Parent Notification and Permission

Informed consent is a critical ethical issue in the implementation of *Reducing the Risk.* Students participating in the program must be aware of what is involved and their **parents must know, in detail, the curriculum content and process** and grant permission for their child to participate.

The recommended steps for parent notification and permission are covered in detail in the section *Prior to Class 1* on page 5.

## Follow District Guidelines

Before teaching this unit the teacher must be certain the program concepts, objectives and approach are within district guidelines and have the full support of the administration, the school board and parents whose children are enrolled in the class.

# PRIOR TO CLASS 1

## INITIATING *REDUCING THE RISK*

### SYNOPSIS

*Reducing the Risk* is designed to be incorporated into a broader family life education program. Before initiating the unit, ground rules for classroom discussion must be established and parent notification and permission for student participation accomplished. Procedures for both are outlined.

### PREPARATION

- Decide how ground rules are going to be presented to students. As necessary, list ground rules on butcher paper for posting, and/or make a copy for each student.
- According to district guidelines, write and copy parent permission letters for distribution at least two weeks prior to teaching any topic of sexuality or this curriculum specifically.
- Begin to prepare for the **Visit or Call a Clinic** assignment in Class 8.
- *Optional:* Have ready *Ground Rules* Poster from *Reducing the Risk Supplementary Kit.*

# TIMELINE

| Activity | Time | Schedule |
| --- | --- | --- |
| Ground Rules | 15 minutes class time | At least one day prior to Lesson 1 |
| Parent Permission | 10–20 minutes class time | At least 2 weeks prior to any lessons about sexuality |

## Ground Rules for Classroom Discussion

To accomplish the goals of this program, students need to feel free to talk about sexuality, birth control and protection from sexually transmitted disease. It is not always easy for students to do so. To create the atmosphere of trust and comfort in which sufficiently detailed discussions can take place, ground rules for classroom discussion should be established.

One option for establishing ground rules is to use the *Guiding Principles or Ground Rules* suggested in this section. These can be posted on the chalkboard or bulletin board and/or copied for each student.

Another method is to elicit the ground rules from students using the Socratic method:

- Ask students to suggest reasons why people might be afraid to speak up in a class that deals with sexuality. Draw such reasons as embarrassment, fear of what others would think, not knowing correct words or terms, appearing to know too much, looking dumb, etc. (*Note:* keep the discussion in terms of other people's fears to allow freer discussion.) List these fears on the board.
- When a reasonable list has been made, ask students for ground rules that would make it more comfortable for everyone to speak freely.
- Generate a list that includes the following:

### Guiding Principles or Ground Rules

1. Everyone has the "right to remain silent" about any thoughts and actions he or she wishes to keep private.

2. Every question is a good question; every comment is worthy of consideration. Questions indicate a desire to learn or to confirm what you suspect. Students who ask the most questions will also learn the most.

3. Teasing, putting down or talking about other class members' comments inside or outside of the classroom is rude and will not be allowed.

4. The teacher will respect the above confidentiality ground rule as well, except when she/he is required by law to disclose information (for example, when a student gives reason to suspect sexual abuse). Confidentiality cannot be maintained if what is shared is illegal or dangerous to you or other students (for example, if a student confides that he or she is using heroin at school).

5. If you or people you know have a concern, complaint or question about the class, discuss it with the teacher as soon as possible.

6. When you discuss the issues raised in class with parents, give an accurate accounting of what the class is about. Try to give specific examples and do not sensationalize.

7. Role plays can be informative and fun if treated seriously in class and forgotten after class. Because role plays are based on a fictional situation, students may say things in the role play that they would not say otherwise. Nothing said in a role play should be considered to indicate an interest in having a relationship or sex.

## Anonymous Question Box *(Optional)*

An anonymous question box provides the opportunity for all students to get answers to questions they might be hesitant to ask in class. It also gives teachers time to think about answers to difficult questions or to look for more information.

To build the box, cut a slit in the lid of a shoebox or other similar box, then tape the lid to the box. Introduce the box to students by displaying it and explaining its purpose. Provide paper for students to write their questions on.

### Tips for Using Anonymous Questions

1. Assure students that all questions will be taken seriously.

2. If you don't know the answer to a question, research it and report back to students.

3. Some questions may be better answered privately. Offer students the option of signing their questions if they want a private, written answer.

# Steps for Parent Notification and Permission

Informed consent is a critical ethical issue in the implementation of *Reducing the Risk.* It is essential that parents know the content and process and grant permission for their child to participate.

Four steps are recommended:

1. Announce *Reducing the Risk* in the semester prior to implementation.

   a. The announcement should be included in a standard form of communication by the principal to the parents.

   b. The announcement should clarify that this is primarily a new approach to teaching family life education as opposed to a new curriculum.

   c. The announcement should express the purpose of the curriculum: to reduce teen pregnancy and STD infection, including HIV, by teaching social skills to successfully result in behavior that will prevent an unwanted and unprotected sexual encounter.

   d. The announcement should precede registration so parents and students will be aware of a change in the family life education course.

2. Students registered for the *Reducing the Risk* class should receive a letter informing them and their parents of the process and content of the program. The letter should:

   a. Describe in detail the content of the curriculum.

   b. Inform parents that they may view the full curriculum at the district/high school office.

   c. Include a permission slip for parental approval or denial of permission to participate.

3. A presentation should be made to students that emphasizes the importance of parent notification and permission.

   a. Explain that the school officials and teachers feel strongly that parents have a right to know and make decisions about their sons' and daughters' education.

   b. Suggest that their parents are people who are very concerned about them as individuals.

c. Ask students to think about what concerns and questions parents might have about sexuality education (e.g., what will be taught, will they teach views consistent with mine, who's the teacher, will this information encourage my child to be sexually active?).

d. If time permits, have two students role-play parents with concerns and questions discussing the course with the teacher.

4. A parent preview should be scheduled to give parents an opportunity to meet the teacher and better understand the rationale and teaching approach used in this curriculum. The meeting could present an overall description of the curriculum, give parents an opportunity to review learning activities and to discuss the homework assignments and the perceived benefits of doing these assignments.

## Prepare for the Class 8 "Visit or Call a Clinic" Assignment

In Class 8, students will be given an assignment to visit or call a clinic. At this time, read the Class 8 section to determine the possible options for this assignment. Well before Class 8 you should begin to learn more about local clinics. To facilitate students' visit to a clinic—which may be the most important single element in the entire curriculum—you will need to know:

1. what clinics in your community are available to handle the students who wish to visit.
2. what the clinics' guidelines are regarding the number of students who can visit at a time.
3. whether appointments are needed prior to visits.
4. how many total students they can serve.
5. the best times to call or answer questions.

Individual visits to the clinic are the most effective for enhancing students' ability to attend a clinic. At some future date if they want birth control or protection, other arrangements can also increase their comfort with going to a clinic. These arrangements, as described in Class 8, are field trips and speakers. If visits to a clinic are not feasible, then one or both of the latter arrangements must be developed before Class 8.

## Using Role Plays

This curriculum moves to the beat of "practice, practice, practice." Students get considerable experience talking to their peers in order to learn to manage situations that might otherwise lead to unprotected sex. Because such situations are, in real space and time, more highly charged than they are in the classroom, students must *overlearn* ways to handle themselves. If they complete the curriculum and are still tentative about what to say and do, then their chances of being clear and forceful in the throes of romance are not great.

Some students and classes see each role play as a new challenge, which is how it was designed. The role plays become more challenging for students as the lessons progress. Others see them each as the same, and after a few role plays their interest ebbs. The *practice* is more important than the way they practice, so teachers should feel free to create alternative ways to role-play. Teachers have reported success with the following approaches:

- Have students write role plays as homework assignments.
- Have students write down responses and then role-play in front of the class.
- Have students generate a list of challenging "lines." Then have a student read the lines to the class and have each student give a response.
- Have students develop and act out plays (that is, longer scripts).

Other ideas will surely emerge as you use this curriculum. For greater detail and step-by-step instructions for how to use role plays see Appendix C.

# CLASS 1

# ABSTINENCE, SEX AND PROTECTION— PREGNANCY PREVENTION EMPHASIS

## SYNOPSIS

Class 1 is an introduction to *Reducing the Risk.* The teacher models two versions of a role play to demonstrate refusal skills. Students participate in a two-part "pregnancy risk" activity to personalize their vulnerability to pregnancy.

## PREPARATION

- Review *Introduction* and *Prior to Class 1* and assure yourself that the Parent Notification and Permission is complete.
- Review Appendix C, "How to Use Role Plays."
- For ease of "performance," copy **Lee and Lee #1** and **#2** (Teacher Role Plays 1.1 and 1.4) so that they are separate from the book.
- Cut out 12 paper squares, number them 1 to 12 and place them in a hat or other container.
- Make a copy of the **Pregnancy Risk Chart** (Teacher Reference 1.3); cut the chart into the 12 numbered strips as marked.
- Starting with the current month, vertically list the names of the next 12 months of the year on the board.
- For each student, copy **My Risks** (Worksheet 1.2).

## OUTLINE OF ACTIVITIES

| Activity | Time | Material |
|---|---|---|
| Introduce Curriculum and Model Role Play, Version 1 | 10 minutes | **Lee and Lee #1** (Teacher Role Play 1.1) |
| Months of the Year Risk Activity, Parts I and II | 25 minutes | **My Risks** (Worksheet 1.2) and **Pregnancy Risk Chart** (Teacher Reference 1.3) |
| Model Role Play, Version 2 | 10 minutes | **Lee and Lee #2** (Teacher Role Play 1.4) |
| Lesson Summary | 5 minutes | None |

### NOTE TO THE TEACHER

Both parts in the introductory role play, **Lee and Lee**, are written to be read by one person—you—for several reasons. This initial presentation sets the tone and breaks the ice for the student role plays that follow, so an adult-modeled first script is important. Performing alone is usually the best approach, since teachers rarely have access to an opposite-sex adult assistant to play the other part, and asking a student to read with a teacher could be misinterpreted.

## ACTIVITIES

### Introduce Curriculum and Model Role Play, Version 1

1. Tell students that today is the beginning of a new unit that will give them skills to keep from getting pregnant or from getting someone else pregnant. To introduce the informational skills they'll be learning, you're going to do a one-person play. The dialogue of the play might now, or in time, be familiar to them.

The play is called **Lee and Lee**. Tell students you'll be playing Lee and also her boyfriend—who is, amazingly, also named Lee. (Ask students to hold their applause until the end!) See **Lee and Lee #1** (Teacher Role Play 1.1). As necessary, change the names of the characters or the language in this role play to work for your students.

2. After you've resumed your role as teacher, ask students their reaction to the way Lee and Lee discussed having sex. Include the following questions in the discussion:

   a. Is this the way many couples decide whether or not to have sex?

   b. Why didn't Lee stick to the decision not to have sex?

   c. What makes it difficult to say no?

Tell students that even though they may know how to avoid pregnancy, and want to, it's not always easy to say no to sex or use protection. It takes *knowledge* and *skills*. The story of Lee and Lee shows that many young people don't have either the knowledge or the skills.

Every year, over 1 million teenagers become pregnant.

Yet, pregnancy is preventable. Tell students this unit helps them do something about the problem of unplanned teen pregnancies. They will learn they can avoid pregnancy by practicing the skills to abstain or use protection. In the next few weeks, they will act out situations like **Lee and Lee** that they may face outside the classroom. After role-playing in class and completing assignments as homework, they will be better prepared to be sure that real-life encounters do not lead to unwanted sex or pregnancy.

## NOTE TO THE TEACHER

The purpose of the Pregnancy Risk activity is to demonstrate the ***substantial*** risk teens have of getting pregnant when they engage in unprotected sex. The activity is not intended to demonstrate specific statistical risk, but to help students personalize their risk of pregnancy and think about how their lives would change if they did get pregnant or get someone pregnant. Therefore, the activity is designed so that *all* students in the class do "get pregnant."

You may want to clarify two things at the end of the activity:

- In real life, it is possible that some students might not experience a pregnancy within a year. However, there is a risk of pregnancy *every* time you have unprotected sex, including the first time. It is also possible to get pregnant more than once in a year.
- Data show that teens who engage in unprotected sex for a year have a 90 percent chance of experiencing a pregnancy within that year. For the purpose of this activity, we are assuming that teens who engage in unprotected sex have a 100 percent chance of pregnancy for that year.

# Pregnancy Risk Activity

## Part I:

1. Tell students this activity will help them understand the risks of having sex without using protection. Explain that a couple has a 1 in 12 chance of a pregnancy each time they have sex. That means almost everyone who has sex once a month will get pregnant in the first year. It doesn't mean that if they have sex 11 times they will not get pregnant. Pregnancy could happen the first time.

2. Write the months of the year on the board, beginning with the current month. Have the container with the numbered squares ready. Pass out **My Risks** (Worksheet 1.2). Ask students to choose a number from 1 to 12 and write it at the top of their worksheet. This will be their number for both parts of the activity.

3. Explain that for purposes of this activity we will make believe that everyone in the class is having unprotected sex once a month, although we know that a large percentage of young people their age are not having sex.

4. Have a student draw a square out of the container and read the number aloud. Write the number beside the first month on the board (which should be the current month). Ask all students who have put that number on their worksheet to stand. When students are standing, tell class that this is how many pregnancies there would be at the end of the first month of unprotected sex. Assure students that you know boys don't get pregnant but they do share equal responsibility in a pregnancy.

5. Ask any of the students standing to either "pass the hat" or write the numbers on the board.

6. Ask another student to draw a number. Write that number beside the second month and ask students with this number to stand. These students would be pregnant at the end of the second month. Continue drawing numbers until all the numbers are gone or all students are standing, whichever comes first. Tell students that they are all pregnant! Remind them that this is based on having sex once a month.

7. Have students sit down. Remind them that the 1 in 12 chance is random. It doesn't mean only getting pregnant the twelfth time a couple has unprotected sex. It can happen the first time.

8. Have students fill out Part A of **My Risks** (Worksheet 1.2). Allow five minutes to complete the worksheet.

9. Ask volunteers to share their responses to some of the immediate results of a positive pregnancy test (e.g., telling your partner [for the girl], parents, friends). Based on when their hypothetical pregnancy would occur, ask for other volunteers to state how that pregnancy would affect their life that year (e.g., Christmas, prom, summer vacation, etc.).

10. Ask students if getting pregnant is just a matter of luck like picking numbers. Draw out in the discussion that they can choose not to get pregnant by using *self-control* and saying no to sex, or using *protection.*

## Part II:

11. The second part of this activity shows how risk changes when people abstain or use protection correctly and consistently. Place the numbered strips from the **Pregnancy Risk Chart** (Teacher Reference 1.3) in the container (hat) and leave the months and numbers from Part I on the board.

12. Ask a student to draw a strip from the container and read the *number only* aloud. Ask students with that number to stand. Then have the student read the rest of the information on the strip. Write "pregnant" or "not pregnant" next to the number on the board. Students may sit down if they are not pregnant.

13. Now ask another student to draw a strip from the container and repeat the process. Continue until all numbers are gone. (In this part of the exercise, most students won't get pregnant at all. Those who do may not get pregnant for many months.)

14. After all the numbers are drawn, ask students to complete Part B of **My Risks** (Worksheet 1.2). Allow three minutes to complete the worksheet.

15. Ask volunteers to share their responses to Part B of the worksheet. Lead a discussion around all the things students can do if they do not have to cope with a pregnancy (finishing the school year, participating on the swim team, earning money after school for a car, etc.). Briefly process with students which "life course" is more desirable.

16. Next, in a guided discussion, ask volunteers to share how they felt about the "pregnancy" (Part I) and what effects a real pregnancy would have on their current lives. Use the following points to help guide the discussion:

- Adoption, abortion or even a pregnancy scare can have serious personal consequences. These can ruin relationships, alienate parents and make their remaining high school years very difficult.
- Researchers believe that teen pregnancy is associated with much lower levels of the three E's: less *education;* less *employment* in well-paying, interesting jobs; and less *enjoyment* of later life. Children born to teenage parents may have a harder time in school and are less likely to be happy, since their parents often pass their problems along.

## Model Role Play, Version 2

1. Return to the story of Lee and Lee. Tell students that this time Lee and Lee will make a different decision because they have participated in a class like this one and now have the skills to say no. They start as before, kissing and touching on the sofa. (Again you assume the role of both Lees.) See **Lee and Lee #2** (Teacher Role Play 1.4).

2. Briefly discuss why version two ended differently than version one. Explain that in the next lesson the class will discuss three reasons that the role plays ended differently.

## Lesson Summary

Remind students this class has introduced them to ideas they'll be studying for the next three weeks:

- Teenagers can and should avoid pregnancy.
- The only sure ways to avoid pregnancy are to abstain (not have sex) or always use protection.
- It's not easy to always follow either of these two courses of action; but
- There are skills for handling situations in ways that are sophisticated, successful (at avoiding pregnancy and keeping relationships) and safe.

# Lee and Lee #1

**NARRATOR**: Lee and Lee have been going out for three months, and, although taking it slow, they've been getting closer to having sex. They're sitting on the sofa together. Music is playing. Lee and Lee begin to get down to some serious kissing and touching.

**Lee**: Don't, Lee. Let's stop.

**Lee**: Why?

**Lee**: I don't know. I don't think I'm ready for this. And we don't have anything to use for protection.

**Lee**: Being ready just means we love each other. You do still love me, don't you?

**Lee**: You know I do, but what if something happened? What about getting pregnant or getting an infection like HIV?

**Lee**: We could handle having a baby. It would look just like you—we could name it Lee. I think that'd be great.

**Lee**: Oh, Lee. I don't know…

**Lee**: Listen, don't worry about getting pregnant. We can stop before anything happens.

**Lee**: I don't think that works…

**Lee**: What do you mean? Tammy's not pregnant, is she? What do you think they use? Besides, we're the lucky types. We found each other, didn't we? How else would two people named Lee get together if somebody wasn't looking out for us?

**Lee**: (Laughs and kisses Lee) I really do love you, Lee. You're right—we're two lucky people.

**Lee**: Ummhhmmm hummhhhh.

**NARRATOR**: Lee and Lee went ahead and had sex without using birth control. Despite Lee's prediction about stopping in time and being lucky, Lee did get pregnant. She had the baby the night of the sophomore dance—but neither Lee nor Lee went to the dance.

# My Risks

My number is ____________.

**Part A.** I (my girlfriend) would be pregnant after just ____ months of having unprotected sex. We would have a baby in the month of ________________ if I (or she) carried the baby to term.

1. Within a few days of finding out about the pregnancy, I would have to:

______________________________________________________________________

______________________________________________________________________

______________________________________________________________________

______________________________________________________________________

2. The pregnancy would change the next year of my life by:

______________________________________________________________________

______________________________________________________________________

______________________________________________________________________

______________________________________________________________________

**Part B.** I don't want to be a teenage parent because I want to:

1. ____________________________________________________________________

____________________________________________________________________

2. ____________________________________________________________________

____________________________________________________________________

3. ____________________________________________________________________

____________________________________________________________________

# Pregnancy Risk Chart

*Directions:* Copy and cut on dotted lines.

1. You did not become pregnant, because you used a latex condom and foam correctly every time you had sex.

2. You did not become pregnant, because you decided not to have sex and you stuck to your decision.

3. You did not become pregnant, because you used a latex condom and foam correctly every time you had sex.

4. You did not become pregnant, because you decided not to have sex and you stuck to your decision.

5. You did not become pregnant, because you decided to use the pill and you (or your girlfriend) took it every day.

6. You did not become pregnant, because you decided to use a condom and foam and used it correctly every time you had sex.

7. You (or your girlfriend) are pregnant because you didn't abstain or use protection.

8. You did not become pregnant, because you told your boyfriend (or girlfriend) you didn't want to have sex and stuck to your decision.

9. You (or your girlfriend) are pregnant because you decided to use condoms but you didn't use one every time.

10. You (or your girlfriend) are pregnant because you didn't abstain or use birth control.

11. You did not become pregnant, because you decided to use the pill and you (or your girlfriend) took it every day.

12. You did not become pregnant, because you decided to use the pill and you (or your girlfriend) took it every day.

# Lee and Lee #2

**Lee**: No, Lee. Stop.

**Lee**: Why?

**Lee**: I'm not ready for this. And besides, if we do it we need to—you know—use something for protection.

**Lee**: Being ready just means we love each other. You do still love me, don't you?

**Lee**: Yes, but being ready means more than that. We're not ready if we don't have protection. I am saying NO to becoming a parent and to HIV.

**Lee**: Nothing's going to happen, Lee.

**Lee**: I know, because we're not going to do anything without using something—no matter how much I love you.

**Lee**: We could handle having a baby. It would look just like you—we could name it Lee. I think that'd be great.

**Lee**: (Laughs) Stop joking, Lee. I'm serious. I have NO plans to become a parent while I'm in high school.

**Lee**: Listen, don't worry about getting pregnant. We can stop before anything happens.

**Lee**: That doesn't work. That's not protection.

**Lee**: What do you mean? Tammy's not pregnant, is she? What do you think they use? Besides, we're the lucky types. We found each other, didn't we? How else would two people named Lee get together if "Lady Luck" wasn't looking out for us?

**Lee**: (Laughs) Well, I traded lockers with Daryl, for one thing, so we'd see each other every day.

**Lee**: You did?

**Lee**: Sure. And then I learned your schedule so I'd happen to run into you a lot. I believe in helping luck along.

**Lee**: You're really something, Lee. You're right about the protection—and besides, I won't do it till it's right for both of us.

**Lee**: C'mon, let's go out and get something to eat.

**NARRATOR**: Lee and Lee leave to get hamburgers. Lee learned a lot about luck from Lee. That was the year Lee got a great after-school job and Lee won a college scholarship.

ALTERNATE

# CLASS 1

# ABSTINENCE, SEX AND PROTECTION— HIV PREVENTION EMPHASIS

## SYNOPSIS

In Alternate Class 1 the teacher models two versions of a role play to demonstrate refusal skills to help prevent HIV infection. Students participate in an "HIV risk" activity to personalize their vulnerability to HIV and to symbolically experience modes of HIV transmission. This class can be substituted for Class 1 or used in addition to Class 1.

## PREPARATION

- Review *Introduction* and *Prior to Class 1* and assure yourself that the Parent Notification and Permission is complete.
- Review Appendix C, "How to Use Roleplays."
- For ease of "performance," copy **Lee and Lee #1H** and **#2H** (Teacher Role Plays 1.1H and 1.3H) so that they are separate from the book.
- For each student, copy **My HIV Risks** (Worksheet 1.2H).
- Have one package each of pink, white, blue and green 3" x 5" index cards. You will need four index cards for each student. Count out 50% pink cards, 25% white, 10% blue and 15% green (e.g., with 40 students [160 cards], count out 80 pink cards, 40 white cards, 16 blue cards and 24 green cards). You will also need two yellow index cards.

## OUTLINE OF ACTIVITIES

| Activity | Time | Material |
|---|---|---|
| Introduce Curriculum and Model Role Play, Version 1 | 10 minutes | **Lee and Lee #1H** (Teacher Role Play 1.1H) |
| HIV Risk Activity | 20 minutes | Index cards, chalkboard |
| Personalizing Risks | 5 minutes | **My HIV Risks** (Worksheet 1.2H) |
| Model Role Play, Version 2 | 10 minutes | **Lee and Lee #2H** (Teacher Role Play 1.3H) |
| Lesson Summary | 5 minutes | None |

### NOTE TO THE TEACHER

Both parts in the introductory role play, **Lee and Lee #1H**, are written to be read by one person—you—for several reasons. This initial presentation sets the tone and breaks the ice for the student role plays that follow, so an adult-modeled first script is important. Performing alone is usually the best approach, since teachers rarely have access to another adult assistant to play the other part, and asking a student to read with a teacher could be misinterpreted.

## ACTIVITIES

### Introduce Curriculum and Model Role Play, Version 1

1. Tell students that today's class will give them skills to keep from getting infected with HIV. Tell students that HIV is the virus that causes AIDS. People who have HIV in their bodies are said to have HIV infection or be HIV-positive. An HIV-positive person can be very healthy or very sick. People with

HIV can pass the virus to their sex partner or to someone they share a needle with even if they do not have symptoms and are unaware of being infectious.

2. Many young people don't have either the knowledge or the skills to prevent getting HIV.

   To introduce the informational skills they'll be learning, you're going to do a one-person play. The play is called **Lee and Lee** (and is similar in format but different in content from the play in Class 1). Tell students you'll be playing Lee and Lee's friend—who is, amazingly, also named Lee. (Ask students to hold their applause until the end!) See **Lee and Lee #1H** (Teacher Role Play 1.1H). As necessary, change the names of the characters or the language in this role play to work for your students.

3. After performing the role play, resume your role as teacher and ask students their reaction to the way Lee and Lee discussed having sex and the risk of HIV. Include the following questions:

   a. Is this the way many teenagers decide whether or not to have sex?

   b. Why didn't Lee stick to the decision not to have sex?

   c. What makes it difficult to say no?

   Tell students that in this unit they will learn skills to prevent HIV. In the next few lessons, they will act out situations like "Lee and Lee" that they may face outside the classroom. After role-playing in class and completing assignments as homework, they will be better prepared to be sure that real-life encounters do not lead to unwanted sex, pregnancy or HIV.

## HIV Risk Activity

1. Tell students that this activity will help them understand how HIV is spread, and the risks of getting HIV.

2. Distribute four cards of one color to each student. Ask students to write their names on each card. Tell students they will be introducing themselves to four other people by exchanging cards. Model this process by exchanging your two yellow cards with those of two students.

3. Inform all other students (except those with white cards) that they now have three minutes to mingle and exchange cards.

4. Explain privately and quietly to the students with white cards that they represent abstinence. The other students should not be able to hear this information. When other students try to exchange cards with them, they are to hold onto their white cards and refuse to exchange them. It is okay for these students to accept cards (representing advances) from other students.

5. Reconvene the whole group. Announce that, for this particular activity, you are HIV-positive and those people with whom you exchanged your yellow cards were exposed to the virus.

6. Explain the meaning of the colors of the other cards:

- People with pink cards had unprotected sex.
- People with blue cards used latex condoms consistently and correctly.
- People with green cards shared needles (to inject drugs or vitamins or for tattooing or piercing).
- People with white cards abstained from risky behaviors.

7. Ask the two students who had contact with the teacher to stand and state who else they had contact with (by reading the names on the cards they collected). Ask the other students to stand when they hear their names called—if they had unprotected sex (pink cards) or shared needles (green cards) with the person calling their name.

8. Illustrate the pattern of transmission by writing on the chalkboard the names of the first two students (yellow cards) and listing their contacts to the right. Ask those who are still sitting to stand if they had "risky" contact (pink cardholders and green cardholders) with any student already standing. Ask everyone to sit down.

9. Ask the students with the white cards to stand. Announce that they represent abstinence, and that many approached them but they used refusal skills to protect themselves.

   Ask these students to sit down.

10. Ask the students:

  a. How did it feel waiting for your name to be called once you learned that the teacher "infected" the two students? (Dispel any anxiety expressed.)

  b. How did you feel about getting HIV?

  c. How did it feel to approach the students with white cards? What refusal skills did they use?

  d. Ask the students with the white cards to share how it felt to refuse contact.

11. Acknowledge that those who originally had blue cards reduced their risk of infection by using latex condoms consistently and correctly.

12. Emphasize that the contacts in this activity symbolized transmission of HIV. The virus is not transmitted through casual contact.

13. Have students fill out Parts A and B of **My HIV Risks** (Worksheet 1.2H). Allow five minutes to complete the worksheet.

14. Ask volunteers to share their responses to some of the immediate results of a positive HIV test (e.g., telling your partner, parents, friends).

15. Ask for other volunteers to state how getting HIV might affect their lives.

16. Then, lead a discussion around all the things students can do if they do not have to cope with getting HIV.

## Model Role Play, Version 2

1. Return to the story of Lee and Lee. Tell students that this time Lee and Lee will make a different decision because they have participated in a class like this one and now have the knowledge regarding HIV prevention and the skills to say no. They start as before, kissing and touching on the sofa. (Again you assume the role of both Lees.) See **Lee and Lee #2H** (Teacher Role Play 1.3H).

2. Briefly discuss why version two ended differently than version one. Explain that in the next lesson the class will discuss three reasons why the role plays ended differently.

## Lesson Summary

Remind students that this class has introduced them to ideas they'll be studying for the next few lessons:

- All of us are at risk for HIV infection depending on what we do. It's not who we are but what we do that places us at risk.
- HIV is mainly transmitted through unprotected sex or needle-sharing with an HIV-infected person.
- For teenagers, abstinence from needle use and sex are the best choices. The second best choice is to use condoms. The third best choice is to avoid having multiple partners.

  In a later lesson they will receive further information about risk situations, HIV transmission, symptoms and prevention.

# Lee and Lee #1H

**NARRATOR**: Lee and Lee have been going together for four months. They're sitting on the couch together.

**Lee**: Don't, Lee. Please, stop.

**Lee**: Why?

**Lee**: I'm scared. We don't have anything to use for...protection.

**Lee**: Don't worry. We don't have anything to worry about.

**Lee**: But what if something happens? What if I get something like HIV?

**Lee**: Don't worry. You wouldn't get HIV. Kids like *us* aren't at risk! It's only hard-core kids that get HIV.

**Lee**: I've been scared of getting HIV for months...ever since you told me you and Ronnie didn't use...well, you know...rubbers. I've heard about Ronnie.

**Lee**: What did you hear?

**Lee**: I heard Ronnie has HIV. That's what everyone is saying at school. I'm scared.

**Lee**: I'm not worried. I don't have anything to worry about. I feel great. I look good, don't I? Besides, I only went out with Ronnie a few times.

**Lee**: It wouldn't matter if it was only once. Anyone who has sex with someone who has HIV can get HIV.

**Lee**: Listen, Lee. We're lucky. How else would two people named Lee get together if somebody wasn't looking out for us? And the only thing that's important is that we have each other.

**Lee**: (Laughs and kisses Lee) You're right—we're two lucky people. I'm crazy about you too, Lee.

**NARRATOR**: Lee and Lee went ahead and had sex without using a condom. Despite their belief about being lucky, Lee was diagnosed HIV-positive shortly before their graduation.

# My HIV Risks

**Part A.** You learn that you may have been infected with HIV.

1. Within a few days of finding out that I might be HIV-infected, I would have to:

____________________________________________

____________________________________________

____________________________________________

____________________________________________

2. If my HIV test showed that I had HIV, I would have to:

____________________________________________

____________________________________________

____________________________________________

____________________________________________

**Part B.** I don't want to become infected with HIV because:

1. ____________________________________________

____________________________________________

2. ____________________________________________

____________________________________________

3. ____________________________________________

____________________________________________

# Lee and Lee #2H

**NARRATOR**: Lee and Lee have been going together for four months. They're sitting on the couch together.

**Lee**: Don't, Lee. Please, stop.

**Lee**: Why?

**Lee**: I'm scared. We don't have anything to use for...protection.

**Lee**: Don't worry. We don't have anything to be concerned about.

**Lee**: But what if something happens? What if we get something like HIV?

**Lee**: Don't worry. We wouldn't get HIV. Kids like *us* aren't at risk! I love you. That's the only thing that matters.

**Lee**: I love you, too. But kids like us *do* get HIV. I heard that Ronnie's got HIV, and I'm scared because you told me you had sex together and didn't use rubbers.

**Lee**: I'm not worried. I feel great. I look good, don't I? Besides, I only went out with Ronnie a few times.

**Lee**: It wouldn't matter that it was only once. Anyone who has sex with someone who has HIV can get HIV.

**Lee**: Listen, Lee. We're lucky. How else would we have found each other? And the only thing that's important is that I'm crazy about you.

**Lee**: Well, maybe we've been lucky in the past. But now I'm scared. I love you too, Lee, but I've decided to wait to have sex.

**Lee**: You're right. We have too much to look forward to, to risk losing everything. Let's go see that new movie that's playing.

**NARRATOR**: Neither Lee nor Lee became infected with HIV. They graduated that June very much in love, looking forward to college.

# CLASS 2

# ABSTINENCE:

# NOT HAVING SEX

## SYNOPSIS

Class 2 reminds students that there are only two ways to avoid pregnancy and HIV—not having sexual intercourse (abstaining), or consistently using protection. This session focuses on the advantages of abstinence. Additionally, reasons why teens fail to abstain or protect are considered. Students also discuss elements of successful male/female communication about abstinence. They practice identifying successful elements of communication in the role play from Class 1.

## PREPARATION

- For each student, copy **Lee and Lee #2** (Worksheet 2.1).
- Write the *Facts About Abstinence* (p. 42) on the board or butcher paper. Leave blanks for the percentages.
- Review **Lee and Lee #2** (Teacher Key 2.2).
- For each student, copy **What Abstinence Means to Me** (Worksheet 2.3).

# OUTLINE OF ACTIVITIES

| Activity | Time | Material |
|---|---|---|
| Review Previous Lesson | 5 minutes | None |
| Communicating About Abstinence | 15–20 minutes | **Lee and Lee #2** (Worksheet 2.1) and **Lee and Lee #2** (Teacher Key 2.2) |
| Facts About Abstinence | 10 minutes | *Facts About Abstinence* on the board |
| Reasons That Many Teens Don't Have Sex | 10 minutes | **What Abstinence Means to Me** (Worksheet 2.3) |
| Lesson Summary | 2 minutes | None |

# ACTIVITIES

## Review Previous Lesson

Ask students what they have learned from the previous lesson(s) about the risk of getting pregnant and/or the risk of HIV infection. (Having sex without protection is high risk; most couples who have unprotected sex will get pregnant, and all couples will risk HIV infection. Students don't have to rely on luck to avoid pregnancy and HIV infection.)

## Communicating About Abstinence

1. Tell students there are many ways to avoid pregnancy and sexually transmitted disease (STD). You could become a hermit (briefly define if necessary) who never talks to anyone or does anything. Or, you could avoid pregnancy and STD by being so unpleasant that everyone stays clear of you. Or you could never become involved in a romantic relationship.

   Ask students to think about whether any of these are good ways to avoid pregnancy, HIV and other STD. Acknowledge they are not, because many people want:

- to have a boyfriend or girlfriend
- to be liked
- to get along with people
- to have a family someday

Tell students that in this unit the class will be talking about how to avoid pregnancy and STD and still have successful relationships.

2. Explain to students that there are three basic elements that provide a foundation for successful romantic relationships. Write the elements on the board, and briefly explain each:
   - Strong honest *communication* (C): being honest and saying what you want so there is no doubt you mean it.
   - *Relationship* building (R): talking and acting in a way that shows you want to keep a good relationship going.
   - *Planning* (P): talking and acting to make your future healthy and happy. Planning shows knowledge of what you want and how to get it.

3. Hand out **Lee and Lee #2** (Worksheet 2.1). Ask students to read the worksheet and underline and identify the places in the dialogue that demonstrate strong communication (C), relationship building (R), and planning (P). Using **Lee and Lee #2** (Teacher Key 2.2) lead the class through the identification process for the first few lines of dialogue. Then let students work on their own. Explain that there may be some lines of dialogue that represent more than one element for building successful relationships. Allow five minutes to complete the worksheet. (*Optional:* Have students work in pairs to identify these elements.)

4. In the full group, briefly process student responses. Discourage them from thinking only about "right" and "wrong" answers. There should be considerable latitude around students' perceptions. The point is for students to understand that you can be strong in your words and actions and still maintain a positive relationship.

5. Summarize that *talking* about love, sex, protection and relationships is critical to getting what you want and avoiding what you don't want. Talking about these things is hard, so it is tempting to just hope that your boyfriend or girlfriend will understand what you want and do it. Teens who are pregnant or got someone pregnant, when asked what they talked about in the situations that led to pregnancy, often say, "We didn't talk about it, we just did

it." Not talking about it will almost surely put you at risk for pregnancy, HIV or other STD.

Tell students that in the next few weeks they will spend a lot of time talking about and practicing what to say and do to avoid pregnancy or HIV and other STD. Abstaining, or not having sex, is one way to keep from getting pregnant or getting a sexually transmitted disease. Next, the class will look at some reasons not to have sex.

## Facts About Abstinence

1. Some people believe that "everyone" is having sex. But there are strong personal, medical and relationship-building reasons for teenagers not to have sex—that is, to abstain from sexual intercourse. Many teens know that. Let's look at the statistics and see the percentage of teens who are saying no to having sex.

2. Refer to the *Facts About Abstinence* statements on the board. For each statement, ask the class for their estimates of the percentages of teens not having sex. Then fill in the blanks with the correct figures. Tell students that these statistics were reported in 1994 (Alan Guttmacher Institute, *Sex and America's Teenagers,* 1994).

### Facts About Abstinence

- At age 15, about _____% (82%) of all young people have not had sex.
- About _____% (48%) of males and _____% (64%) of females under 17 report never having had sex.
- Nearly _____% (20%) of adolescents do not have sex at all during their teenage years.

# Reasons That Many Teens Don't Have Sex

1. Tell students that, as they know, some young people do have sex. Ask them to think about likely results of having sex. List their results on the board, adding any important factors they miss. Students may include some positive outcomes (e.g., "It's fun" or "It makes us feel close") and these should be acknowledged as reasons that millions of teens risk getting pregnant, or infected with HIV and other STD each year. Indicate in this discussion that each of these positive reasons can make it difficult for males and females who choose not to have sex to stick with their choice. Also, discuss whether the positive responses are always true. Ask what circumstances make them true or not true.

2. Next, ask students to help you brainstorm a list of personal, psychological and medical reasons that make abstaining from sex a valid option. As each reason is identified, write it on the board, butcher paper or an overhead transparency. Encourage students to identify reasons to abstain from sex for *now* or for the next few years, perhaps until marriage. A nearly comprehensive list of reasons follows. Use it to add to or embellish the reasons students suggest.

   - Many young people believe in and practice abstinence for *religious* reasons and personal *moral* beliefs.
   - Abstinence can be a sign of real *emotional maturity* and *integrity.* Many young women and men report feeling pressured into having sex before they are ready. It requires maturity and honesty to resist the pressure of someone you love in order to make a decision that is consistent with personal values, morals and needs.
   - Abstinence *reduces* the risk of getting sexually transmitted diseases such as herpes, chlamydia, gonorrhea and HIV. We will discuss these more in a later session.
   - Abstinence is the only method of birth control that is *100 percent effective,* 100 percent safe and 100 percent free of side effects.
   - Abstinence reduces the risk of cervical cancer. Research suggests there is a connection between early sexual activity, multiple sexual partners and increased cervical cancer in women under age 25.
   - Abstinence shows that you are stronger than peer pressure.
   - Many parents would be hurt and upset to know that their child is having sex. This may spoil a couple's relationship.

- A couple may find that delaying sexual intercourse contributes in a positive way to their relationship. Abstaining may allow them time to *develop a deeper friendship.* They may spend more time talking, building mutual interests, sharing good times with other friends and establishing an intimacy that is other than sexual.
- Abstaining can be a *test of love.* Counter to the old line "You would if you loved me," not having sex can allow time to test the endurance of love beyond the first attraction and before having sexual intercourse.
- Abstaining may contribute to teaching people to be *better lovers;* it allows them to explore a wide range of ways to express love and sexual feelings.

3. To personalize this information, hand out **What Abstinence Means to Me** (Worksheet 2.3). Ask students to think about the likely results of not having sex and to complete question 1. Ask volunteers to read their responses. (If appropriate, add new ones to the list on the board.) Ask them to add to their list results they hear from other students or from you. When students identify negative outcomes, acknowledge that there are strong pulls away from abstaining that will be considered throughout the unit. Students should then complete question 2.

## Lesson Summary

Acknowledge that it is sometimes hard to practice abstinence. A good way to respond to the "It's hard to remain abstinent" message is to return to the advantages of not becoming pregnant or HIV-infected, and to note that abstinence is often a way to do what's safest and "right" for you. (Explain to students that if it doesn't seem like the right time for sex, it probably isn't.)

# Lee and Lee #2

*Directions:* Write ***C*** when you see strong *Communication* statements and underline them. Write ***R*** when you see *Relationship-Building* statements and underline them. Write ***P*** when you see *Planning* statements and underline them.

**Lee**: No, Lee. Stop.
**Lee**: Why?

**Lee**: I'm not ready for this. And besides, we would need to use something for protection and we don't have it.
**Lee**: Being ready just means we love each other. You do still love me, don't you?

**Lee**: But being ready means more than love. We're not ready if we don't have protection. I am saying no to getting pregnant and to HIV.
**Lee**: Nothing's going to happen, Lee.

**Lee**: I know, because we're not going to do anything without using something—no matter how much I love you.
**Lee**: We could handle having a baby. It would look just like you—we could name it Lee. I think that'd be great.

**Lee**: (Laughs) Stop joking, Lee. I'm serious. I have no plans to be a parent while I'm still in high school.
**Lee**: Listen, don't worry about getting pregnant. We can stop before anything happens.

**Lee**: That doesn't work. That's not protection.
**Lee**: What do you mean? Tammy's not pregnant, is she? What do you think they use? Besides, we're the lucky types. We found each other, didn't we? How else would we have gotten together if "Lady Luck" wasn't looking out for us?

**Lee**: (Laughs) Well, I traded lockers with Daryl, for one thing, so we'd see each other every day.
**Lee**: You did?

**Lee**: Sure. And then I learned your schedule so I'd happen to run into you a lot. I believe in helping luck along.
**Lee**: You're really something, Lee. You're right about the protection—and besides, I won't do it till it's right for both of us.

**Lee**: C'mon, let's go out and get something to eat.

**NARRATOR**: Lee and Lee leave to get hamburgers. Lee learned a lot about luck from Lee. That was the year Lee got a great after-school job and Lee won a college scholarship.

# Lee and Lee #2

*Directions:* Write ***C*** when you see strong *Communication* statements and underline them. Write ***R*** when you see *Relationship-Building* statements and underline them. Write ***P*** when you see *Planning* statements and underline them.

**Lee**: No, Lee. Stop. (**C**)
**Lee**: Why?

**Lee**: I'm not ready for this. (**P**) And besides, we would need to use something for protection and we don't have it. (**C & P**)
**Lee**: Being ready just means we love each other. You do still love me, don't you?

**Lee**: But being ready means more than love. We're not ready if we don't have protection! (**C**) I am saying no to getting pregnant and to HIV. (**P**)
**Lee**: Nothing's going to happen, Lee.

**Lee**: I know, because we're not going to do anything without using something—no matter how much I love you. (**C** & **R**)
**Lee**: We could handle having a baby. It would look just like you—we could name it Lee. I think that'd be great.

**Lee**: (Laughs) Stop joking, Lee. I'm serious. I have no plans to be a parent while I'm still in high school. (**P**)
**Lee**: Listen, don't worry about getting pregnant. We can stop before anything happens.

**Lee**: That doesn't work. That's not protection. (**C**)
**Lee**: What do you mean? Tammy's not pregnant, is she? What do you think they use? Besides, we're the lucky types. We found each other, didn't we? How else would we have gotten together if "Lady Luck" wasn't looking out for us?

**Lee**: (Laughs) Well, I traded lockers with Daryl, for one thing, so we'd see each other every day. (**R**)
**Lee**: You did?

**Lee**: Sure. And then I learned your schedule so I'd happen to run into you a lot. I believe in helping luck along. (**R**)
**Lee**: You're really something, Lee. You're right about the protection—and besides, I won't do it till it's right for both of us.

**Lee**: C'mon, let's go out and get something to eat. (**R**)

**NARRATOR**: Lee and Lee leave to get hamburgers. Lee learned a lot about luck from Lee. That was the year Lee got a great after-school job and Lee won a college scholarship.

# What Abstinence Means to Me

1. *What are the advantages to me if I don't have sex at this time in my life?*

   a. ______________________________

   ______________________________

   b. ______________________________

   ______________________________

   c. ______________________________

   ______________________________

   d. ______________________________

   ______________________________

2. *What makes it difficult not to have sex?*

   a. ______________________________

   ______________________________

   b. ______________________________

   ______________________________

   c. ______________________________

   ______________________________

   d. ______________________________

   ______________________________

# CLASS 3

## REFUSALS

### SYNOPSIS

Class 3 includes a discussion of the student/parent homework assignment. The teacher introduces verbal and nonverbal communication skills. Students are provided with a demonstration of the social skills important to abstaining and using protection. They are also given the chance to practice and examine the five characteristics of effective refusals.

### PREPARATION

- Review Appendix C, "How to Use Role Plays."
- Review Appendix D, "Skills Overview."
- Make copies of homework **Talk to Your Parents** (Homework 3.1) (2 pages).
- Write the *Refusals* (p. 53) on the board or butcher paper OR have ready *Refusals* Poster from *Reducing the Risk Supplementary Kit (optional).*
- Make two copies of the role plays:
  **Your Friend's Ex-Girlfriend**, Ineffective Version (Role Play 3.2),
  **Your Friend's Ex-Girlfriend**, Effective Version (Role Play 3.3),
  **Trying to Slow Down**, Ineffective Version (Role Play 3.4),
  **Trying to Slow Down**, Effective Version (Role Play 3.5).
- For each student, copy **Observer Checklist** (Form 3.6).
- *Optional:* Have ready *Role Play Cards* from *Reducing the Risk Supplementary Kit.*

# OUTLINE OF ACTIVITIES

| Activity | Time | Materials |
|---|---|---|
| Review Previous Lesson | 5 minutes | None |
| Talk to Your Parents | 15 minutes | **Talk to Your Parents**, Part A and **Talk to Your Parents**, Parts B and C (Homework 3.1) |
| Introduce Refusals | 10–15 minutes | *Refusals* Poster *(optional)* |
| Demonstrate Role Plays | 10–15 minutes | **Your Friend's Ex-Girlfriend** (Role Plays 3.2 and 3.3) and **Trying to Slow Down** (Role Plays 3.4 and 3.5) **Observer Checklist** (Form 3.6) *Role Play Cards (optional)* |
| Lesson Summary | 2 minutes | None |

# ACTIVITIES

## Review Class 2

Review the following from the previous lesson:

- Abstinence is more common than most people think.
- Reasons for abstinence.
- Three parts of a successful relationship.

## Talk to Your Parents

1. Hand out **Talk to Your Parents**, Part A (Homework 3.1). Explain that this homework involves two distinct sections. Part A is for students to complete and asks for their ideas about sex and protection. In addition, Part A asks students to indicate what they *think* their parents believe about the same things. Have students complete Part A in class.

2. Distribute Part B and assign interviews to be turned in by Class 6. Let students know that the benefit of the homework comes from talking and listening to parents; therefore, they should not just give the sheet to their parents to fill out. Tell students that their parent interview is completely confidential and they will *not* turn in the homework. Instead, to verify that the homework was completed, the student and parent will sign a form stating that they did the assignment. This form is the only thing the student will turn in.

## Introduce Refusals

### NOTE TO THE TEACHER

> The class will briefly discuss verbal and nonverbal aspects of effective refusals and then see how the skill can be put into practice. This class demonstrates the skill of refusals and also familiarizes students with the routine of role-playing and using observer checklist forms to note how the skill was used.

### Verbal Refusals

1. It is sometimes hard to say no—especially to someone we care about—and to stick with it. Sometimes we're saying no, but it doesn't come across as NO. Tell students they will use a series of role plays to learn about, and then practice, ways to say no when they don't want to have sex. The ability/skill to say no effectively gives us a lot of power over our lives.

2. Provide a quick overview of the refusals model students will be using. List the five behaviors on the board or display the *Refusals* Poster from the Supplementary Kit. (See Appendix D, "Skills Overview," for specific examples of each refusal behavior.)

> **Refusals**
>
> 1. Say "No!"
> 2. Repeat the refusal.
> 3. Suggest an alternative.
> 4. Use body language that says "No!"
> 5. Build the relationship (if appropriate).

3. Refer to the three elements of successful relationships (communication, relationship building, planning) and point out how refusal statements can fit with these elements. Emphasize that the verbal aspect of effective refusals involves saying the word *no* in a tone of voice that shows you mean it, repeating the refusal if necessary, and suggesting an alternative. You can also reinforce the verbal refusal in nonverbal ways.

### Nonverbal Refusals

4. Explain that "body language" (such as tone of voice, gestures, the look on your face, the way you sit or stand) is an important way to communicate with or without talking. Ask the class to describe body language that says no to sex. Generate a list like the one below. Write the list on the board and demonstrate each behavior to reinforce the concept of nonverbal communication.

    a. **Hands off**—throwing hands up in a "get off of me" gesture or using hands for emphasis.

    b. **Soldier body**—sit up or stand up stiffly like a soldier at attention and march away from the other person if you need to.

    c. **Firm voice**—strong and business-like voice.

    d. **Serious expression**—best "I mean it" face.

    e. **Gestures**—hand and arm movements that emphasize point.

    f. **Fight back**—at times, if everything else fails, you might have to use your strength to push away and protect yourself.

## Demonstrate Role Plays

1. The role plays **Your Friend's Ex-Girlfriend** (Role Plays 3.2 and 3.3) and **Trying to Slow Down** (Role Plays 3.4 and 3.5) demonstrate some of the ways that *not clearly saying no* can work against getting what you want. Pass out the role plays and **Observer Checklist** (Form 3.6) to all students. Ask them to listen and watch the role plays and check off the behaviors that are used during each role play. Or, assign observers a specific behavior to watch for in the role play. For example, one group of observers looks for "Said No," another for "Repeated Refusal," etc.

2. Preselect a male and a female student to read the role plays. Begin with **Your Friend's Ex-Girlfriend**, Ineffective Version (Role Play 3.2). You should read the "Setting the Stage" section of the

role play. After the role play is read, conduct a discussion. Ask role players to comment on how they felt in the role and how they would feel if this were a real situation. Ask students to identify what the guy did or did not do that led to his ineffectiveness. Pull for such ideas as:

- He never said no.
- He never repeated his first objection.
- He was trying not to upset the girl and did not use clear communication.
- He expressed doubt and left her thinking it might work out.

3. Then have the same two students read **Your Friend's Ex-Girlfriend**, Effective Version (Role Play 3.3), keeping the same roles. Again the teacher should read the "Setting the Stage" section of the play. After the role play, thank the participating students and ask them to sit.

4. Have two new students read the ineffective version of **Trying to Slow Down** (Role Play 3.4). Have students use the checklist to record the use of effective refusals after the role play. Review the use of refusals with students. Help them recognize that Person 2:

   - never said no
   - never restated the first objection
   - asked questions ("Do you love me?") rather than stating her or his view
   - expressed doubt
   - failed to offer any alternative actions
   - failed to use "hands off" or other body language
   - gave up

5. Now have the same students read the effective version of **Trying to Slow Down** (Role Play 3.5), keeping the same roles. Have students use the checklist. Discuss the elements of Person 2's effective refusal.

## Lesson Summary

Conclude by reminding students that today they practiced and observed clear refusal statements that tell a person they mean no without losing a friendship. Remind students that the skills they are learning can be used in a variety of situations.

# Talk to Your Parents

Part A

*Directions:* Fill in the blanks on Part A with your own ideas, including how you think your parent(s) would answer. Then talk to your parent(s) and see how close you are. Record their answers on Part B of this form.

1. How should teenagers show affection to someone they love?

   What I think: ______________________________

   ______________________________

   What I think my parent(s) think: ______________________________

   ______________________________

2. Should adolescents have sex with someone they love if they plan to marry them?

   What I think: ______________________________

   ______________________________

   What I think my parent(s) think: ______________________________

   ______________________________

3. What are the best kinds of protection for teenagers who are sexually active?

   What I think: ______________________________

   ______________________________

   What I think my parent(s) think: ______________________________

   ______________________________

4. What should parents do to help their child avoid pregnancy or HIV infection?

   What I think: ______________________________

   ______________________________

   What I think my parent(s) think: ______________________________

   ______________________________

# Talk to Your Parents

Part B

1. How should teenagers show affection to someone they love?

   What my parent(s) do think: ______________________________

   ______________________________

2. Should adolescents have sex with someone they love if they plan to marry them?

   What my parent(s) do think: ______________________________

   ______________________________

3. What are the best kinds of protection for teenagers who are sexually active?

   What my parent(s) do think: ______________________________

   ______________________________

4. What should parents do to help their child avoid pregnancy or HIV infection?

   What my parent(s) do think: ______________________________

   ______________________________

Due date:______________________

- - - - - - - - - - - - - - - - - - - - - - - - - - - - - -

Part C

We verify that we completed the **Talk to Your Parents** homework assignment.

______________________________ Parent's or Guardian's signature

______________________________ Student's signature

# Your Friend's Ex-Girlfriend

Ineffective Version

*Setting the stage:*

Your best friend's girlfriend broke up with him. Now she seems very interested in going out with you. You like her, but you really don't want to go out with her because you have been going out with another girl and don't want to mess it up. She speaks first.

**Girl**: I haven't seen you for a while. Let's go out some night.

**Guy**: Well, I don't know.

**Girl**: I just want to talk to you about some things.

**Guy**: Call me sometime, it gets boring at home.

**Girl**: Let's go check out a movie. We could go this weekend.

**Guy**: I may be busy.

**Girl**: I know we'd have fun together.

**Guy**: I suppose.

**Girl**: I'll give you a call this weekend. Maybe we can do something? OK?

**Guy**: I guess so. See ya.

# Your Friend's Ex-Girlfriend

Effective Version

*Setting the stage*:

Your best friend's girlfriend broke up with him. Now she seems very interested in going out with you. You like her, but you really don't want to go out with her because you've been going out with another girl and don't want to mess it up. She speaks first.

**Girl**: I haven't seen you for a while. Let's go out some night and do something fun.

**Guy**: I miss you, too, but I'm interested in someone else right now.

**Girl**: I just want to talk to you about some things.

**Guy**: I don't want to lead you on, but I'd be glad to talk.

**Girl**: Let's go check out a movie. We could go this weekend.

**Guy**: Sorry. I've already got plans to go out.

**Girl**: What about next Saturday night?

**Guy**: No, I really don't want to go out.

**Girl**: I guess we're not going to be friends, huh?

**Guy**: Well, I'd like to be friends, I just don't want to go out.

# Trying to Slow Down

Ineffective Version

*Setting the stage:*

You and your boyfriend (girlfriend) have been going out for a while. From the beginning you touched and kissed a lot. On his (her) birthday, you are alone and feel very close. After you have had something to celebrate the birthday, you begin kissing and touching and feeling really good. Your boyfriend (girlfriend) wants to have sex with you, but you decide to tell him (her) that you are not ready.

**Person 1**: Why are you stopping now?

**Person 2**: Wait. I'm not sure that I'm ready.

**Person 1**: It isn't my birthday every day, you know.

**Person 2**: Yeah, I know.

**Person 1**: There's no reason to wait. It will mean even more now. What's the difference, now or later?

**Person 2**: Well, I'm not sure.

**Person 1**: I thought this was what we both wanted.

**Person 2**: Do you love me?

**Person 1**: Yes, and sex is part of love.

**Person 2**: I guess you're right.

(They stop talking and go back to kissing)

# Trying to Slow Down

Effective Version

*Setting the stage:*

You and your girlfriend (boyfriend) have been going out for a while. From the beginning you touched and kissed a lot. On her (his) birthday, you are alone and feel very close. After you have had something to celebrate the birthday, you begin kissing and touching and feeling really good. Your girlfriend (boyfriend) wants to have sex with you, but you decide to tell her (him) that you are not ready.

**Person 1**: Why are you stopping now?

**Person 2**: This feels good, but let's not have sex now.

**Person 1**: It isn't my birthday every day, you know.

**Person 2**: Yeah, I know, but I don't think we're ready.

**Person 1**: I've never had sex and want to have it with you first.

**Person 2**: Maybe some day, but, no, not now.

**Person 1**: There is no reason to wait. It will mean even more now. What's the difference, now or later?

**Person 2**: I want to wait.

**Person 1**: I thought this was what we both wanted.

**Person 2**: We both want to be close, but I don't want sex. How about opening your present from me? It's in my backpack.

**Person 1**: OK.

Name: ______________________________ Date: ______________________________

# Observer Checklist
## Refusals

ROLE PLAY #

| BEHAVIOR | 1 | 2 | 3 | 4 | 5 | 6 |
|---|---|---|---|---|---|---|
| Said "NO" | | | | | | |
| Body Language Said "NO" | | | | | | |
| Repeated Refusal | | | | | | |
| Suggested Alternative | | | | | | |
| Built the Relationship | | | | | | |

# CLASS 4

## USING REFUSAL SKILLS

### SYNOPSIS

Class 4 quizzes students on refusal skills and uses role plays to practice using these new skills in difficult situations.

### PREPARATION

- Review Appendix C, "How to Use Role Plays."
- Review Appendix D, "Skills Overview."
- For each student, copy **Refusals** (Quiz 4.1).
- Make two copies of the scripted version of **At a Party** (Scripted Role Play 4.2).
- For each student, have a copy of **At a Party** (Role Play 4.3).
- For each student, copy **Observer Checklist** (Form 4.4).
- *Optional:* Have ready *Role Play Cards* from *Reducing the Risk Supplementary Kit.*

# OUTLINE OF ACTIVITIES

| Activity | Time | Materials |
|---|---|---|
| Refusals Quiz | 10 minutes | **Refusals** (Quiz 4.1) |
| Difficult Refusals | 5 minutes | None |
| Demonstrate Role Play | 5 minutes | **At a Party** (Scripted Role Play 4.2)<br>**Observer Checklist** (Form 4.4) |
| Role-Play in Small Groups | 15–30 minutes | **At a Party** (Role Play 4.3)<br>**Observer Checklist** (Form 4.4)<br>*Role Play Cards (optional)* |

# ACTIVITIES

## Refusals Quiz

1. Distribute **Refusals** (Quiz 4.1). Allow five minutes for students to complete.

2. Have students correct their own papers. Discuss each statement, asking volunteers to describe why it does or does not meet the guidelines for a clear refusal statement.

3. Ask students to recall the five characteristics of an effective refusal statement. List them on the board.

## Difficult Refusals

1. Tell students that you want their ideas about things their friends might say to them that make saying no more difficult. Ask them to get out a piece of paper and write one or two "lines" that boys or girls they know might use to convince them to do something they don't want to do—cut a class, lend them their nicest clothes, go out somewhere, have sex or have unprotected sex. Suggest a couple of lines. For example, "You would if you loved me" or "Try it, you'll like it!" Give them a few minutes to complete responses to the lines.

2. In the full group, read the lines. Have volunteers share effective responses to each statement. Use several lines on one student to show how they can just repeat the refusal over and over without having to think up new lines.

## Demonstrate Role Play

1. Recruit students to act out both parts of the script **At a Party** (Scripted Role Play 4.2). Explain that they will need to pay attention to the verbal and nonverbal skills as they watch the actors. Give them a copy of the **Observer Checklist** (Form 4.4) to use to indicate which behaviors the actors used. Or, assign observers a specific behavior to watch for in the role play.

2. After actors have read and demonstrated the role play, ask them how they felt about their roles. Review the skills that were used. Ask observers for examples of:

   - saying no
   - body language that said no
   - repeated refusals
   - suggesting an alternative
   - relationship building

## Role-Play in Small Groups

1. Explain to students that they will be working in small groups on role plays. In their group they will be rotating through various roles. Each student will have the opportunity to read a script (scripted role), respond to a script (unscripted role) and watch (observer).

   Pass out the role play **At a Party** (Role Play 4.3). At their seats, give students no more than five minutes to write down what they might say in the role play to avoid unprotected sex when they have the unscripted part. They can use these responses to help prepare for the role play, although they should not just read when they do the role play. They should act as if this is a real scene and they have no script to rely on—they have to rely on themselves.

2. Have students divide into groups with a mixture of males and females. Students should bring their role plays and ideas for responses to the group.

*Optional:* Pass out a set of *Role Play Cards* to each group. Ask each member to take one card. Review each role with the whole group. Write key words on the board:

- Student Role Player #1: Read lines.
- Student Role Player #2: Respond to lines.
- Student Observer #1: Set the stage for the role play, and use **Observer Checklist** (Form 4.4).
- Student Observer #2: Use **Observer Checklist** (Form 4.4) and lead small group discussion using the guidelines on the back of the card.

3. Make sure each student still has an **Observer Checklist** (Form 4.4). Instruct students to alternate within the group, reading the script and playing in the unscripted role. After a student reads the script, that student takes the unscripted role. Make sure each student has the chance to participate in both the scripted and the unscripted roles and to provide observer comments. The observer is the person who is next in order to read the script.

If the groups do not have equal numbers of boys and girls, then have them assume the other role so everyone has the opportunity to participate in both roles. If there is time to go around a second time, the script readers can repeat the script or choose to ad-lib and make up their own lines.

## NOTE TO THE TEACHER

It is important to help groups "get going" with the role plays. It may be necessary for the teacher to designate who in each group will start the scripted and unscripted roles and to guide the role-play process.

During the role plays, walk around the room to assess how students are using the skill. You may offer coaching if students are stuck or are using the skill incorrectly.

Time each round of practice and tell students when to pass their cards for the next round. Once students become more familiar with this type of practice, you can allow each group to monitor the rounds.

4. When groups are finished, have students return to the full group and discuss the experience. Explain that their comfort working like this in small groups will increase each day as the process is repeated throughout the unit.

   Use the following points to guide discussion:

   - Identify feelings that came up about using the skill during the practice. What was easy? What was difficult?
   - Discuss how this situation was or wasn't similar to real life.
   - Discuss any barriers to using the skill. Have students identify ways to overcome these barriers.
   - Ask what left the biggest impression as a result of the role play.
   - Ask students to identify how they will use the skill in the next week with their friends.

# Refusals

1. Write one statement for each of the following that includes at least two elements of an effective refusal.

   a. C'mon, you don't have to go home yet. It's not that late. Your mom will understand.

   ______________________________________________

   ______________________________________________

   ______________________________________________

   b. You've said you love me. Now I want to show you that I love you—let's make love.

   ______________________________________________

   ______________________________________________

   ______________________________________________

2. Put a check mark beside statements that follow at least one guideline for effectively saying no.

________ a. No, I don't trust you.

________ b. Well, I don't know. Probably not.

________ c. No, thanks. I don't want to go to that party. Why don't we go to the movies instead?

________ d. Why don't you go ask someone else?

________ e. I don't think we should be doing this.

________ f. No, not now. Let's watch TV instead.

________ g. But you promised you wouldn't ask me that.

# At a Party

*Setting the stage:*

You are at a party with someone you have gone out with a few times. The party is at somebody's home and their parents are gone. A lot of kids are getting high and some couples are leaving—maybe to have sex. You don't want to have sex and don't want to leave the party.

**Person 1:** Let's get out of here so we can talk—it's too crowded.

**Person 2:** Yes, it is crowded in here—but the porch is empty.

**Person 1:** I just want to be with you. This is our chance.

**Person 2:** I want to be with you, too, but the party's fun.

**Person 1:** C'mon, I just want to be alone with you.

**Person 2:** No, I like this party—I'm glad we came.

**Person 1:** I've been looking forward to this night with you—please don't spoil it.

**Person 2:** I hope the night won't be spoiled.

**Person 1:** If I'd known you'd be like this, I wouldn't have come here with you.

**Person 2:** I guess not, but I know we can have fun. Let's get something to eat in the kitchen.

**Person 1:** I guess I don't have much choice.

**Person 2:** Yes, I suppose so. But I'll give you the choice of the next movie we go to.

# At a Party

*Setting the stage:*

You are at a party with someone you like and have gone out with a few times. The party is at a friend's house and their parents are gone. A lot of kids are getting high and some couples are leaving—maybe to have sex. You don't want to have sex and don't want to leave the party. Your date speaks first.

**Person 1**: Let's get out of here so we can talk—it's too crowded.

**Person 2**:

**Person 1**: I just want to be with you. This is our chance.

**Person 2**:

**Person 1**: I've been looking forward to this night with you—please don't spoil it.

**Person 2**:

**Person 1**: If I'd known you'd be like this, I wouldn't have come here with you.

**Person 2**:

**Person 1**: I really thought you were going to be a lot of fun.

**Person 2**:

**Person 1**: Don't worry. I'm not going to do anything. C'mon, let's go.

**Person 2**:

Name: ______________________ Date: ______________________

# Observer Checklist
# Refusals

ROLE PLAY #

| BEHAVIOR | 1 | 2 | 3 | 4 | 5 | 6 |
|---|---|---|---|---|---|---|
| Said "NO" | | | | | | |
| Body Language Said "NO" | | | | | | |
| Repeated Refusal | | | | | | |
| Suggested Alternative | | | | | | |
| Built the Relationship | | | | | | |

# CLASS 5

## DELAYING TACTICS

### SYNOPSIS

Class 5 introduces delaying tactics. Students observe the teacher demonstrate and practice delaying skills in role-play situations. A short quiz at the end of the lesson reviews delaying.

### PREPARATION

- Review Appendix C, "How to Use Role Plays."
- Review Appendix D, "Skills Overview."
- Write the *Delaying Tactics* (p. 87) on the board or butcher paper OR have ready *Delaying Tactics* Poster from *Reducing the Risk Supplementary Kit (optional).*
- For each student, copy **Possible Delaying Tactics** (Handout 5.1).
- For each student, copy **Presents and Flowers** (Role Play 5.2).
- For each student, copy **Observer Checklist** (Form 5.3).
- For each student, copy **Refusing or Delaying Quiz** (Quiz 5.4).
- *Optional:* Have ready *Role Play Cards* from *Reducing the Risk Supplementary Kit.*

# OUTLINE OF ACTIVITIES

| Activity | Time | Materials |
|---|---|---|
| Review Class 4 | 5 minutes | None |
| Introduce Delaying Tactics | 20–40 minutes | **Possible Delaying Tactics** (Handout 5.1)<br>*Delaying Tactics* Poster *(optional)* |
| Demonstrate and Practice Role Play in Small Groups | 5–15 minutes | **Presents and Flowers** (Role Play 5.2)<br>**Observer Checklist** (Form 5.3)<br>*Role Play Cards (optional)* |
| Quiz and Skills Review | 10–20 minutes | **Refusing or Delaying Quiz** (Quiz 5.4) |
| Lesson Summary | 2 minutes | None |

# ACTIVITIES

## Review Class 4

Review the elements of an effective refusal.

## Introduce Delaying Tactics

1. Explain that *delaying tactics* are another way to handle difficult situations and avoid unwanted and unprotected sex. For many reasons, it's usually better to simply say no to offers you don't like. But people often feel confused about how to say no. Others may not have the courage to say no to their friends. Without time to think of what to do, they can impulsively make a poor decision. In such cases people might use a delaying tactic to gain time to think about what they really want. Remember, sooner or later you have to give a clear no message.

2. Provide an overview of the delay model students will be using. List the five behaviors on the board or display the *Delaying Tactics* Poster from the Supplementary Kit. It is important to point out that an effective delay doesn't need to use all these behaviors. The goal is to end the interaction as quickly as possible and not let it drag on.

(See Appendix D, "Skills Overview," for specific examples of each delaying tactic.)

> **Delaying Tactics**
>
> 1. Make a delay statement.
> 2. Take a delay action.
> 3. Create space.
> 4. End the situation quickly.
> 5. Build the relationship (if appropriate).

3. Pass out **Possible Delaying Tactics** (Handout 5.1). Briefly review the examples and ask students to add additional statements and actions.

## Demonstrate and Practice Role Play

Use the same format for role play as described in Class 4. Pass out **Presents and Flowers** (Role Play 5.2) and the **Observer Checklist** (Form 5.3) to each student.

a. Allow the students to write responses that Person 2 could use. Ask them to try to apply one or two of the delaying tactics.

b. Have two students demonstrate the role play.

c. Divide into groups with at least two males and two females in each group.

d. Students should count off in the groups and rotate scripted, unscripted and observer roles. Tell students they don't have to repeat *Setting the Stage* each time they enact the role play. Once they understand the setting they can go directly to the dialogue. The Observers should look for behaviors that show delaying tactics. It is not necessary to use all the tactics to be effective.

*Optional:* Pass out a set of *Role Play Cards* to each group. Ask each member to take one card. Review each role with the whole group. Write key words on the board.

- Student Role Player #1: Read lines.
- Student Role Player #2: Respond to lines.
- Student Observer #1: Set the stage for the role play, and use **Observer Checklist** (Form 5.3).
- Student Observer #2: Use **Observer Checklist** (Form 5.3) and lead small group discussion using the guidelines on the back of the card.

## Quiz and Skills Review

Give out **Refusing or Delaying Quiz** (Quiz 5.4). After students complete it, have them exchange papers with the student next to them. Go over the content to review the skills.

## Lesson Summary

Remind students that this class introduced delaying tactics and refusals to help students in situations in which they feel pressured to have sex or do something else they may not want to do. Students probably already use these skills to manage situations with friends and family. Their use to avoid pregnancy, HIV and other STD may be the most important one of all.

# Possible Delaying Tactics

*Directions:* Review the delaying tactics listed below. In the space provided, add additional ones you think of.

**1. Delay Statements**

Things you could *say:*

I'm not ready.
Not now.
Sorry, I have to go.
It's not the right time.
Not tonight—I've got a sore throat.
I have to call home.

______________________________

______________________________

**2. Delay Actions**

Things you could *do:*

Chew a cough drop.
Look distracted.
Drop something.
Stop kissing.
Go to the restroom.
Pretend you lost something.

______________________________

______________________________

**3. Creating Space**

Things you could say or do:

"I need to go think about this."
Arms in front of body.
Take a step back.
Turn away.

______________________________

______________________________

**4. Ending the Situation Quickly**

Things you could say or do:

"I've got to go now."
"Wow, look at the time!"
Push the person away.
Walk away.

______________________________

______________________________

**5. Building the Relationship**

Things you could say:

"I know this isn't easy for you."
"I like you too."
"I'll call you tomorrow."
"I want you to stop."

______________________________

______________________________

# Presents and Flowers

*Setting the Stage:*

You've been seeing someone older for a month. He/she has treated you to dinner and the movies, has driven you places, and buys you presents and flowers. You have really enjoyed all the attention. During a party at your friend's house, he/she suggests that you leave the party and go somewhere private. Your date's body language shows that he/she wants to have sex with you. You do not want to have sex. Your date speaks first.

**Person 1**: Look at all the great things we've done together. I've been so good to you. C'mon, let's go be alone together.

**Person 2**:

**Person 1**: It's no big deal, it's just part of going out.

**Person 2**:

**Person 1**: I just want to be close to you.

**Person 2**:

**Person 1**: Everybody else is doing it—they just don't tell you.

**Person 2**:

**Person 1**: If you really loved me, you would.

**Person 2**:

**Person 1**: I love you, but you don't seem to care about me.

**Person 2**:

Name: ____________________ Date: ____________________

# Observer Checklist
# Delaying Tactics

ROLE PLAY #

| BEHAVIOR | 1 | 2 | 3 | 4 | 5 | 6 |
|---|---|---|---|---|---|---|
| Used Delay Statement | | | | | | |
| Used Delay Action | | | | | | |
| Created Space | | | | | | |
| Ended the Situation Quickly | | | | | | |
| Built the Relationship | | | | | | |

Name ______________________________

# Refusing or Delaying Quiz

1. Write three delaying actions you could use or alternatives you could suggest if you were alone with your boyfriend or girlfriend and wanted to avoid sexual intercourse.

   a. ______________________________

   b. ______________________________

   c. ______________________________

Read the situations below and write the refusal or delaying response you would use to handle the situation. Decide whether to use a refusal or a delaying statement and include an alternative action.

2. Your girlfriend or boyfriend has been drinking and tries to talk you into going for a ride. You don't think you should go but you don't want to get into an argument. You say and do:

   Refusal or delay: ______________________________

   ______________________________

   Alternative action: ______________________________

   ______________________________

3. You're at home with your girlfriend or boyfriend. Your parents will be gone for several hours. You do not want to have sex, but your girlfriend or boyfriend begins to kiss you and tries to take off your clothes. You say and do:

   Refusal or delay: ______________________________

   ______________________________

   Alternative action: ______________________________

   ______________________________

# CLASS 6

# AVOIDING HIGH-RISK SITUATIONS

## SYNOPSIS

Through a class discussion and a mini-lecture, students discover situations termed "yellow alert" and "red alert," situations that can lead to unwanted or unprotected sex. Students practice dealing with the two types of alerts in the activity **Handling Crisis Situations**. Then, using the worksheet **Protection: Myths and Truths** they begin activities related to protecting themselves from pregnancy or HIV and other STD.

## PREPARATION

- Review **Signs of Sex, Signs of Caution** (Teacher Reference 6.1).
- For each student, copy **Handling Crisis Situations** (Worksheet 6.2).
- For each student, copy **Protection: Myths and Truths** (Worksheet 6.3).
- *Optional:* Have ready *Signs of Sex, Signs of Caution* Posters from *Reducing the Risk Supplementary Kit.*

# OUTLINE OF ACTIVITIES

| Activity | Time | Materials |
|---|---|---|
| Discuss Homework | 15 minutes | Completed **Talk to Your Parents** (Homework 3.1) |
| Signs of Sex and Caution Mini-lecture | 10 minutes | **Signs of Sex, Signs of Caution** (Teacher Reference 6.1) *Signs of Sex, Signs of Caution* Posters *(optional)* |
| Handling Crisis Situations | 10 minutes | **Handling Crisis Situations** (Worksheet 6.2) |
| Protection: Myths and Truths, Round 1 | 10 minutes | **Protection: Myths and Truths** (Worksheet 6.3) |

# ACTIVITIES

## Discuss Homework

1. Discuss **Talk to Your Parents** (Part B), from Class 3. Remind students that you don't want them to repeat what their parent(s) said about any question and that they should keep in mind a parent's privacy. Ask them what they learned from *each* question regarding the following issues:

   a. Did your parent(s) answer the way you thought they would?

   b. Did the ideas of your parent(s) give you any different ideas?

   c. Will you talk to your parent(s) about this again? (If not, whom can you talk to?)

   d. Did you or your parent(s) disagree about any question? If so, how did the discussion turn out?

2. As you guide the discussion, keep in mind that the purpose is to encourage students and their parents to talk. Help students listen to the point of view of their parents. Ask them to report what they learned rather than to evaluate whether they agree with their parents. Ask them to turn in the signed sheet to show they completed the assignment.

# Signs of Sex and Caution Mini-Lecture

1. Remind students that there are two ways to avoid pregnancy and HIV infection: say no to sex, or use protection. To be successful at either, you have to GET READY *NOW.* Many teens who get pregnant or infected say they didn't protect themselves because they didn't expect to have sex. In one recent study, two-thirds of teens who had sex without protection said it "just happened." Tell them there are signs they can watch for that will alert them that sex could happen.

   Ask students to think of the signs in two categories: *yellow alert* and *red alert.*

2. *Yellow alerts* are signals that there may be an unprotected "sex crisis" in the future and that you should slow down and prepare yourself to avoid pregnancy or infection. *Yellow alert* signals occur when you:

   a. are not yet with the boy or girl

   b. think that he or she might be thinking about sex

   c. think that there will be a chance for sex because you will be alone

   d. wonder what will happen

   Yellow alert signals tell you that you had better develop a *sound plan* for avoiding having sex, getting pregnant or becoming infected. You may notice yellow alert signals long before the time that you are seeing the boy or girl. For example, you may notice that you are being especially careful about the clothes you pick out, or especially anxious about what you will say and do, or maybe you can't wait to get to school, or you wear something different or special to school or out at night. If you know what *your* signs are and watch for them, you will have enough time to act and avoid unwanted sex, pregnancy or HIV infection. If you miss the signs, you will not.

3. *Red alert* signs show that there is going to be an unprotected "sex crisis" at any moment and you have to act fast to avoid it. *Red alert* signs usually occur about 20 minutes to an hour before the crisis when:

a. You are alone with the boy or girl.

b. You may have done a lot of touching and feeling close.

You can still stop and decide not to have sex or you can still use protection. But if you go past a red alert signal without stopping and/or preparing first, your life may be forever changed.

4. List "Yellow Alert" and "Red Alert" headings on the board and offer a few examples of signs (see Teacher Reference 6.1). Then add signs that the students suggest.

   *Optional:* Display the *Signs of Sex, Signs of Caution* Posters from the Supplementary Kit. Discuss the signs listed. You may want to add student suggestions to the posters or on a separate piece of paper.

5. Lead students in a discussion that focuses on what to do to avoid unwanted or unprotected sex. Use signs offered by students to shape the discussion.

## Handling Crisis Situations

1. Explain to students that they now have had the opportunity to clearly identify sex alert situations. The next step is to learn to deal effectively with those situations. That is, they need to think about possible ways to get out of an alert situation.

2. Distribute **Handling Crisis Situations** (Worksheet 6.2). Students should name two yellow alert signs and two red alert signs and identify an alternative action plan for each. Tell students that red alert situations usually require *alternative actions, delaying* or *refusal* until the crisis passes or until you are able to get protection. In yellow alert situations, students can avoid the situation entirely or get protection so that a red alert situation doesn't occur.

3. Discuss an example: If the student wrote "I get dressed up in my sexiest clothes" as a yellow alert sign, he or she might generate an alternative action plan such as:

   a. I'm going to think through what I will do to stop if I get close to having sex.

b. I'll plan something to do that will keep us away from having sex.

c. I'll stop and get protection at the drugstore before I see him or her.

Allow students to work alone or with one other person to finish the worksheet.

NOTE TO THE TEACHER

> Students may find this exercise difficult, as specificity and planning do not come easily. But it should get students started in planning to avoid an unwanted pregnancy or HIV infection.

4. When students have finished, review each statement and have several volunteers share their suggestions for ways to handle the situation. Remind students that because we are all individuals, some approaches will feel more personally comfortable than others.

## Protection: Myths and Truths, Round 1

1. At some time in their lives, most people decide they are ready to have sex but not to become a parent. To have sex but not become a parent or become infected with an STD, people must consistently and effectively use protection. To do that, they must know what they are doing. This activity helps students learn how much they know and how much they need to know to avoid pregnancy or HIV and other STD.

2. Introduce this activity by explaining there are many myths or nontruths about protection. Tell students they will be involved in a two-part activity designed to help clear up the myths and get the facts about protection.

3. Pass out **Protection: Myths and Truths** (Worksheet 6.3) and have students complete only the Round 1 section. Explain that

they will be completing the Round 2 section after a discussion about protection in a future class. At that time each myth will be reviewed and discussed. Ask students to hand in their worksheets with their names on them to be passed out again for Round 2, which will be done in Class 9. The Teacher Key for **Protection: Myths and Truths** is provided for Round 2.

NOTE TO THE TEACHER:

Depending on the emphasis you bring to teaching this curriculum, your students may not have covered all the material in the *Protection: Myths and Truths* activity. Items related to pregnancy prevention and HIV prevention are all, nonetheless, included in this exercise because all of this material is of interest to youth and relevant to the dual goals of the curriculum.

## Lesson Summary

Conclude the class by reviewing each activity. First students discussed what they learned about their parents. Then they looked at situations that could lead to teenagers becoming involved in an unprotected "sex crisis." These situations were labeled "yellow alert" or "red alert." Students practiced dealing with the sex alert situations to avoid an unprotected sex crisis. Finally, they had the chance to write down what they think about protection facts.

# Signs of Sex, Signs of Caution

## Yellow Alert Signs

△ I get dressed up to look really sexy.
△ I plan to get some beer to help us loosen up.
△ I think about ways to be alone with him or her.
△ I think about touching him or her.
△ We touch "by accident."
△ We talk about being alone at home.

## Red Alert Signs

▲ We make and take chances to touch.
▲ We touch each other in more ways and are getting excited.
▲ We play sexy music.
▲ We go to a place to "get away from everybody."
▲ We are drinking and touching.
▲ We are alone at home.

Name ______________________________

# Handling Crisis Situations

*Directions:* Write down two yellow alert signs. Then describe a plan to prevent or manage the crisis. Then do the same for red alerts.

***YELLOW*** 1. ________________________________________

________________________________________

Alternative Action Plan: ________________________________________

________________________________________

***YELLOW*** 2. ________________________________________

________________________________________

Alternative Action Plan: ________________________________________

________________________________________

***RED*** 1. ________________________________________

________________________________________

Alternative Action Plan: ________________________________________

________________________________________

***RED*** 2. ________________________________________

________________________________________

Alternative Action Plan: ________________________________________

________________________________________

Name ______________________________

# Protection: Myths and Truths

*Directions:* Read each situation and circle ***T*** if you think it's true or ***M*** if you think it's a myth under the Round 1 column. Do not make any marks under Round 2 column until directed to do so.

| | *Round 1* | *Round 2* |
|---|---|---|
| 1. The best way to use a condom is to pull it on tight. | T or M | T or M |
| 2. Teenagers can obtain birth control pills from family planning clinics and doctors without permission from a parent. | T or M | T or M |
| 3. Girls can get pregnant if the penis doesn't actually enter the vagina. | T or M | T or M |
| 4. Using a latex condom correctly every time you have sexual intercourse is very effective in preventing HIV infection. | T or M | T or M |
| 5. Girls can get pregnant if they have sex during their periods. | T or M | T or M |
| 6. Birth control pills used alone are effective in preventing sexually transmitted disease (STD). | T or M | T or M |
| 7. Douching after sex will wash out the sperm and protect against pregnancy and STD. | T or M | T or M |
| 8. A woman is protected from pregnancy the day she begins taking the pill. | T or M | T or M |
| 9. Abstinence is the most effective method of avoiding HIV infection. | T or M | T or M |
| 10. Condoms are effective because they don't break easily and they don't leak. | T or M | T or M |
| 11. Sharing needles to inject drugs is one way to get HIV. | T or M | T or M |
| 12. If a guy pulls his penis out of a girl in time (before he ejaculates), he can be sure to prevent pregnancy. | T or M | T or M |
| 13. Pregnant women who are infected with HIV can pass it on to the baby before it is born. | T or M | T or M |

# CLASS 7

# GETTING AND USING PROTECTION—I

## NOTE TO THE TEACHER

When making decisions about discussing and demonstrating methods of protection from pregnancy and STD, you must **adhere to district guidelines and policies** that may be in effect. Additionally, you must use your best judgment about the appropriateness of these activities in your individual school. Make sure parents have been informed if demonstrations of methods of protection will take place in class.

Throughout the discussion about protection, remind students that this information is for when they decide to have sex, which might not be for a long time. However, it is important information that they will need eventually.

## SYNOPSIS

Chapter 7 uses lectures and demonstrations to provide information on methods for protection against unplanned pregnancy or STD. As a homework assignment, students research prices and descriptions of nonprescription products.

## PREPARATION

- Review the information in *Ways to Prevent Pregnancy—Teacher Notes.*
- For each student, copy two **Shopping Information Forms** (Homework 7.1)
- Have female reproductive chart available *(optional).*
- Have a cloth or paper towel available.
- For visual aids, obtain:
    - three condoms—one lubricated, one nonlubricated with a reservoir tip, one that is coated with spermicide
    - contraceptive foam

### NOTE TO THE TEACHER

In the past, nonoxynol-9 has been recommended for use as a spermicide coating for condoms. Nonoxynol-9 kills sperm, and, in laboratory studies, nonoxynol-9 kills HIV in a test tube. It is not clear, however, whether nonoxynol-9 is helpful in preventing HIV infection in people because further research is needed. Some people are allergic to nonoxynol-9 and may experience skin irritation when using products that contain it. If an allergic reaction happens, it could make HIV transmission *more* likely. People who experience allergic reactions should avoid using products that contain nonoxynol-9.

## OUTLINE OF ACTIVITIES

| Activity | Time | Materials |
|---|---|---|
| Ways to Prevent Pregnancy—Lecture/ Demonstration | 30 minutes | *Ways to Prevent Pregnancy—Teacher Notes* |
| Shopping Information | 10 minutes | **Shopping Information Form** (Homework 7.1) |
| Lesson Summary | 5 minutes | None |

## ACTIVITIES Ways to Prevent Pregnancy—Lecture/Demonstration

1. Tell students you're going to review different methods people use to keep from getting pregnant. Some of the following information will explain statements on the **Protection: Myths and Truths** worksheet. Tell students they'll get a chance to use any new information when they do Round 2 of that activity. Remind students to listen and take notes, because there will be a quiz at the beginning of Class 9.

2. Tell students there are many ways to try to prevent pregnancy. Elicit from students the methods they are familiar with.

   Explain that in this class they will discuss the methods they are most interested in and which are most effective if used correctly or consistently. Emphasize that some methods help prevent both pregnancy and STD, while other methods do not.

### NOTE TO THE TEACHER

The following lecture information is for you, the teacher. Be sure any information and demonstrations for students conform to district guidelines.

## Ways to Prevent Pregnancy—Teacher Notes

**CATEGORIES OF BIRTH CONTROL METHODS**

A. Methods that don't work: withdrawal, douching, "hoping," rhythm.

B. Methods that are very effective if used correctly and consistently every time: abstinence, birth control pill, Norplant, Depo Provera, condom used together with foam.

A. **Methods that don't work:** withdrawal, douching, hoping and rhythm do not work as birth control methods.

1. **Withdrawal:** When a couple has sex, the man takes his penis out of the woman's vagina before he ejaculates (comes) so that his sperm doesn't go into her body. Withdrawal can't be counted on to prevent pregnancy because the man has a few drops of semen on the end of his penis as soon as it becomes erect. Even if he withdraws before he ejaculates, sperm can get

INFORMATION FOR TEACHERS

into the woman's body and make her pregnant or transmit an STD, including HIV. Couples should not rely on withdrawal since it requires them to interrupt sex exactly when they don't want to.

2. **Douching:** After having sex, the woman immediately washes out her vagina hoping to wash out and kill the sperm. Sperm travel very quickly and some will already have moved through the cervix and into the uterus by the time the woman is able to douche. Once the sperm are inside, it's too late.

3. **Hoping:** Hoping you won't get pregnant or believing that "It can't happen to me" doesn't work. One study of teenagers found that half of first pregnancies occur in the first six months after couples begin having sex. One out of five occur in the first 30 days. Sometimes people think that if they have sex once and don't get pregnant, they can't get pregnant. However, just because a woman doesn't get pregnant the first time, or the twentieth time, doesn't mean she won't get pregnant the next time.

4. **Rhythm:** A woman keeps track of her past menstrual cycles and tries to figure out the days when she is least likely to become pregnant—the "safe" days to have sex.

   The rhythm method is likely to fool you into thinking you are safe when you are not. Since sperm live from three to five days, it can be easy for girls to get pregnant when they think they are safe—even during the menstrual period. No woman can really know what will happen in her next cycle, especially young women, because their cycles have different lengths. Illness, stress or fatigue can upset the hormone system and cause ovulation to occur at an irregular time.

NOTE TO THE TEACHER

> There are very effective birth control methods based on the rhythm system: Natural Family Planning, the Billings Method, the Fertility Awareness Method. These require training in proper use, careful record keeping, daily temperature reading, checking cervical mucus, and commitment from both partners. For most young people, these methods are too difficult to use.

B. **Methods of birth control that are very effective if used correctly and consistently:** abstinence, the birth control pill, Norplant, Depo Provera, the latex condom used together with foam.

1. **Abstinence:** Not having sexual intercourse is the safest, simplest, most effective, easiest-to-get method to avoid pregnancy and STD. Abstinence is free, goes anywhere you want to take it, never wears out, and parents (or anyone else) never have to find out that you are using it!

   *Risks and disadvantages:*

   a) There are no health risks at all.

b) The only risk is that someone you like will not agree with you that abstinence is the best choice.

*Advantages and effectiveness:* Abstinence is the safest, most effective way to avoid pregnancy and sexually transmitted disease.

2. **The birth control pill:** Birth control pills contain different amounts of the female hormones estrogen and progesterone. The pill mimics the hormones of pregnancy and stops the woman's body from ovulating.

To use birth control pills, a woman needs to plan ahead. She cannot get and use pills the same day she decides she wants them. First, she has to make an appointment with a doctor or clinic for a pelvic exam and Pap test. After the exam, the doctor or clinician will give her a prescription for the pill and instructions on when to begin taking them. The woman takes one pill at approximately the same time every day. After taking her first pack of pills, she is protected against pregnancy all day, every day, as long as she continues to take a pill every day. The hormones in the pill keep her body from releasing an egg. Without an egg, the woman can't get pregnant.

*Risks and disadvantages:* Because of health risks associated with the pill, women who use the pill must be medically supervised and have regular check-ups at least once a year. The main risk with birth control pills has to do with the circulatory system—blood clotting problems, heart attacks and strokes. These serious problems occur in only a small number of users. Women who smoke or are very overweight or who have health problems such as high blood pressure or diabetes are at much greater risk for these serious side effects and should not use birth control pills.

Minor side effects may include nausea, sore breasts, slight weight gain, skin problems and/or depression. These side effects usually go away after about three months.

The birth control pill alone is not a method of protection against sexually transmitted disease. To prevent STD, condoms must be used in addition to the pill.

*Effectiveness:* The birth control pill is very effective (97% to 99.9%) if the woman:

a) doesn't forget to take it

b) uses other protection during the first month

c) doesn't take someone else's pills

*Advantages:*

a) Some women find the pill to be a convenient form of birth control that does not affect spontaneity.

b) A woman's periods may be lighter, shorter and more regular with less cramping when she takes the pill.

c) The pill may protect a woman from other problems such as pelvic inflammatory disease (PID), ovarian and endometrial cancer and benign breast lumps.

**3. Norplant:** Artificial hormones contained in tiny capsules are placed under the skin of the arm by a clinician. The capsules slowly release hormones into the bloodstream. Norplant stops ovaries from releasing an egg each month. It thickens the mucus in the cervix so it is hard for sperm to enter the womb.

*Risks and disadvantages:* For the first few months, there may be spotting between periods, light periods, longer periods or no period at all. Norplant does not provide any protection against HIV and other STD. Minor surgery is required to insert or remove capsules. The beginning costs can be expensive.

*Effectiveness:* More than 99% effective.

*Advantages:* Norplant can stay in for five years. It can be removed at any time, allowing the woman to become pregnant right away. It is always in place and does not interfere with sex.

**4. Depo Provera:** Depo Provera contains artificial hormones that are injected by a clinician. It stops the ovaries from releasing an egg each month. It thickens the mucus in the cervix so it is hard for sperm to enter the womb.

*Risks and disadvantages:* There are few serious problems for most women. However, it should not be used by women with liver disease, heart disease, breast cancer or blood clots. It may increase the risk of breast cancer. The injection must be provided by a health care provider. Depo Provera may cause heavy periods, irregular periods, light periods or eventually no period at all. It may produce weight changes, moodiness, headaches or dizziness. The woman may not be able to get pregnant for several months after shots are discontinued. It provides no protection against HIV and other STD.

*Effectiveness:* More than 99% effective.

*Advantages:* Depo Provera does not interfere with sex. Injection lasts three months. It can often decrease bleeding and cramping associated with periods. It is safe to use while breastfeeding.

**5. The latex condom:** This is a thin sheath made of fine latex rubber that fits over the erect penis. Condoms are also called rubbers or prophylactics. **Skin condoms (made from sheep membrane) are not as reliable for the prevention of some diseases, including HIV.**

The condom fits snugly over the erect penis and catches the semen when the man ejaculates (comes) so the sperm doesn't enter the vagina. Using condoms correctly means during every instance of sexual intercourse using a new latex condom with spermicide, leaving space at the tip of the condom, putting the condom on before the penis touches the vagina, and carefully taking the penis out after sex. Some condoms are designed with room at the tip. These are called reservoir tip condoms. Plain tip condoms do not have extra room at the tip.

Condoms are available at any drugstore or family planning clinic. They may also be available in outdoor or all-night condom vending machines. Anyone can buy condoms, regardless of age, and no prescription is needed.

*Risks and disadvantages:*

a) There are no serious health risks.

b) A few people find that condoms irritate the skin. Using another brand can solve the problem.

c) Some people complain that the condom reduces sexual feeling. Others find that it makes no difference.

d) Some people complain that they don't like to stop to put the condom on.

e) Some people complain they are allergic to latex and/or the spermicide.

*Effectiveness and advantages:*

a) If a condom is used correctly together with foam (see below) every time a couple has sex, the combined method will work almost all of the time to prevent pregnancy.

b) Condoms often make sex last longer because they make the penis a little less sensitive.

c) Latex condoms help protect against STD, including HIV.

d) Condoms may help prevent cancer of the cervix in women.

e) Condom use is a good way for a man to share in the responsibility for preventing an unplanned pregnancy.

f) With practice, condoms become easier to use. Condom use can become a regular part of a relationship.

6. **Spermicides—contraceptive foam, jelly, cream, suppositories and film:** These are available without a prescription at any drugstore or family planning clinic. There is no age limit for purchasing, and either partner can buy them. Foam is inserted into the vagina each time the couple has sexual intercourse. The foam covers the cervix. Spermicidal agents kill any sperm that try to enter the uterus.

   Foam comes in a can and looks and feels like shaving cream. It is inserted with a special applicator much like a tampon applicator. One full applicator of foam is inserted deep into the vagina near the cervix less than one hour before sexual intercourse. If more than one hour goes by, more foam must be inserted. Since there is no way to tell when the can is almost empty, a couple should keep an extra can of foam on hand.

   Contraceptive jelly, cream, suppositories and film are also available. Like foam, these are inserted into the vagina each time the couple has sexual intercourse.

   *Risks and disadvantages:*

   a) There are no serious health risks associated with spermicides.

   b) You have to insert them just before sex.

   c) You may have to wait a few minutes for some spermicides to become effective. Read the instructions on the container.

d) Some people may have an allergic reaction or skin irritation. The couple can try another brand.

e) Spermicides alone may not prevent HIV infection.

*Effectiveness and advantages:*

a) If foam or another spermicide is used every time with a latex condom, the combined method works almost all of the time as a birth control method.

b) Foam and other spermicides used alone are fairly effective at preventing pregnancy (79–94%) if used correctly and every time.

c) Foam, jelly, cream, suppositories or film, like condoms, are good methods for people who don't have sex on a regular basis because they are used only when needed.

## Shopping Information Homework

1. Tell students that knowing the facts about protection is important. Protection takes more than knowing to avoid pregnancy and STD—it takes action. Hand out two copies of the **Shopping Information Form** (Homework 7.1) to each student and introduce the assignment. Explain that they do not have to buy condoms or foam, but they do need to go to two stores to get prices and descriptions of these items. The homework assignment, due in a later class, gives students the experience of preparing to obtain protection.

2. Tell students to fill in all information for three kinds of condoms and one type of foam. The brand name is the maker of the product. For condoms, also indicate whether the product is lubricated, has nonoxynol-9, and has a reservoir or plain tip. After students leave the store, they should complete items 3 and 4 to indicate how comfortable they were there and whether they would recommend the store to a friend. Put down the store's hours, too, because it may be important to know where to get protection at some odd hours.

## Lesson Summary

Conclude this lesson by stating that there are different methods of protection, each with its own characteristics, disadvantages and advantages. Except for abstinence, there is no 100 percent safe and effective method. Certain methods that are used to prevent pregnancy still require the use of condoms to prevent STD. In the next lesson, Class 8, students will receive specific information on a number of ways to protect against HIV.

# Shopping Information Form

1. Name of store ______________________________________________

2. What protective products are sold here? (List three kinds of latex condoms and one kind of foam and the prices for each product. Indicate the types of condoms you saw.)

| Product | Brand Name | Price | Lubricated? | Nonoxynol-9? | Reservoir (R) or Plain (P) |
|---|---|---|---|---|---|
| Condom: | | | Yes No | Yes No | R P |
| Condom: | | | Yes No | Yes No | R P |
| Condom: | | | Yes No | Yes No | R P |
| Foam: | | | | | |

3. How comfortable would you be buying protection here?

| 1 | 2 | 3 | 4 |
|---|---|---|---|
| very comfortable | fairly comfortable | somewhat uncomfortable | very uncomfortable |

4. Would you recommend that a friend buy protection here? Yes No

Write two sentences telling why or why not.

______________________________________________

______________________________________________

______________________________________________

______________________________________________

______________________________________________

______________________________________________

5. What are the store's hours of business? ______________________

# CLASS 8

# GETTING AND USING PROTECTION—II

## NOTE TO THE TEACHER

When making decisions about discussing and demonstrating methods of protection from pregnancy and STD, you must **adhere to district guidelines and policies** that may be in effect. Additionally, you must use your best judgment about the appropriateness of these activities in your individual school. Make sure parents have been informed if demonstrations of methods of protection will take place in class.

Throughout the discussion about protection, remind students that this information is for when they decide to have sex, which might not be for a long time. However, it is important information that they will need eventually.

## SYNOPSIS

The first half of Class 8 continues with a discussion and visual demonstration of prevention methods, specifically for preventing HIV.

In the second part of Class 8, students prepare to locate clinics in their area and make plans for contacting one to get information about protection.

Students then apply their knowledge about protection to decide which method(s) might be best for them. Options for this lesson include a guest speaker from a local clinic or a field trip to a local clinic.

## PREPARATION

- For visual aid, obtain one latex condom.
- Review information contained in this lesson in *Latex Barriers for Preventing HIV and STD Infection—Teacher Notes.*
- Determine the activities to use in this class based on the most appropriate way to work with your local clinic(s).
- Have a local telephone directory (or several) available.
- For each student, copy **Visit or Call a Clinic** (Homework 8.1).
- For each student, copy **The Way to the Clinic** (Homework 8.2).
- For each student, copy **How Will You Avoid Pregnancy?** (Worksheet 8.3).
- For each student, copy **How Is HIV Infection Prevented?** (Handout 8.4).

## OUTLINE OF ACTIVITIES

| Activity | Time | Materials |
|---|---|---|
| Barrier Methods for Prevention—Lecture/Demonstration | 15 minutes | *Latex Barriers for Preventing HIV and STD Infection—Teacher Notes*<br>1 latex condom |
| Visit or Call a Clinic | 10 minutes | **Visit or Call a Clinic** (Homework 8.1)<br>**The Way to the Clinic** (Homework 8.2) |
| How Will You Avoid Pregnancy? | 10 minutes | **How Will You Avoid Pregnancy?** (Worksheet 8.3) |
| How is HIV Infection Prevented? | 5 minutes | **How Is HIV Infection Prevented?** (Handout 8.4) |
| Lesson Summary | | None |

## ACTIVITIES

# Barrier Methods for Prevention Lecture/Demonstration

Tell students that you're going to discuss and review prevention methods specifically for HIV.

NOTE TO THE TEACHER

> The following lecture information is for you, the teacher. Be sure any information and demonstrations for students conform to district guidelines.

## Latex Barriers for Preventing HIV and STD Infection—Teacher Notes

Latex barriers such as condoms provide a physical and/or chemical shield against HIV. They also protect against other common STD (sexually transmitted disease)—gonorrhea, syphilis, chlamydia and herpes.

**Condoms**

Condoms made of latex provide good protection from HIV when used correctly and consistently during anal, vaginal or oral sex. Spermicides may offer some protection, but their effectiveness in actual use is still uncertain.

*How condoms prevent HIV transmission:*

Latex condoms are effective in preventing HIV infection when they are used properly and consistently. **Condoms made from sheep membranes ("skin" condoms) do not provide the same degree of protection as latex condoms.**

Condoms only provide effective protection against HIV when they are used correctly every time. Condoms must be used from start to finish during every act of anal, vaginal or oral intercourse.

*When buying condoms:*

a) Make sure the condom is made of latex.

b) Make sure the condom has FDA (Food and Drug Administration) approval. The label or box must say the condoms are for "STD prevention" or "disease prevention." Some novelty condoms, like those that glow in the dark, are not meant for disease or pregnancy prevention.

c) Check the expiration date on the condom package. If they are out of date, the condoms should not be used.

*When storing condoms:*

a) Do not expose condoms to heat, sunlight or ozone.

b) Do not store in a wallet, pocket or car glove compartment.

*When condoms don't work:*

The rate of breakage of condoms ranges from 0.6% to 6% during vaginal intercourse. Most condom failures probably result from incorrect use. Condoms can be broken or damaged during sexual activity by:

a) being torn with fingernails, jewelry or other sharp objects during unwrapping

b) being ripped or broken because of pulling instead of rolling onto the penis

c) being pulled too tightly with no room left at the tip

d) use of oil-based creams or lubricants

Condoms work best when used with water-based lubricants, spermicidal foam or jelly, or lubricating jelly (e.g. K-Y jelly). Some condoms are prelubricated.

*When using condoms:*

a) Open the package carefully.

b) Determine which way the condom unrolls but do not unroll the condom before putting it on.

c) Hold the tip of the condom to squeeze out air and leave some extra room for the semen.

d) Put the condom on the end of the erect penis before there is any contact between the penis and the vagina, anus or mouth. While still holding the tip, unroll the condom onto the penis all the way down to the pubic hair. Do not pull at the condom while unrolling it.

*After sex:*

a) Pull the penis out immediately after orgasm.

b) Hold onto the rim of the condom and pull the penis away from the partner. This prevents any spillage of semen.

c) Remove the condom from the penis and throw it away. (Condoms should never be reused.)

**The Role of Spermicides**

Spermicides are chemicals that kill sperm and bacteria.

Spermicides work best for pregnancy prevention when used with condoms. There is evidence that spermicides can help prevent transmission of gonorrhea and chlamydia during vaginal sex; however, the U.S. Centers for Disease Control (CDC) has stated that no data indicate that spermicides make condoms more effective in protecting against HIV infection.

**When to Use Latex Barriers**

It is strongly recommended that latex barriers be used in vaginal sex, anal sex and all oral sex. The purpose is to avoid the mixing of any fluids vaginally, anally or orally. A latex barrier in the form of a condom or latex dam should be used to cover genitalia during *every* sexual encounter.

**INFORMATION FOR TEACHERS**

# Visit or Call a Clinic

1. Explain that many people—including adults—avoid going to a clinic or doctor to discuss protection because they don't know what to expect. Besides learning what services are offered at local family planning clinics, this homework assignment asks students to rate their comfort level while at the clinic. Hand out the two-page homework and tell students they can complete the assignment in one of four ways:

   a. They can visit a clinic, complete homework and describe the way to get to a clinic.

   b. They can visit a clinic and complete homework.

   c. They can call a clinic, complete homework and describe the way to get to a clinic.

   d. They can call a clinic and complete homework.

   Whichever version of the assignment students choose, they must all complete **Visit or Call a Clinic**. For additional points, they may complete **The Way to the Clinic**.

   Pass out a local phone directory (or several) and have students find the clinic section in the yellow pages. Select two or three conveniently located clinics (or the clinics that have agreed to participate) from which they can choose. Have them choose in class so you can control the number of students contacting each clinic. (If there is only one clinic, consider the alternatives below.)

   Have students write the name of their clinic in the space provided on the worksheet. If the clinics have given you information about the best times to answer questions, etc., share those with students. As a general rule, encourage them to visit the clinic in pairs, but discourage going in groups larger than three. Encourage students to go with their boyfriends or girlfriends, even those who aren't in the class. Tell students they should bring back some literature available from the clinic. This could be a pamphlet or a flier describing services. Remind them that clinics are professional places and that they should use their best behavior. Additionally, they should keep to themselves the names of anyone they see at the clinic.

2. Conduct a brainstorming session to generate some questions that can be used when visiting the clinic.

   If students are slow getting started, help them prepare to ask:

   a. How much does a clinic visit cost?

   b. What is the confidentiality policy?

c. What services are available?

d. How long does it take to get an appointment?

e. Do you have to want a method of protection now, or can you make an appointment for a consultation only?

f. What happens during a typical appointment and how long does it take?

g. Does the clinic also offer HIV testing? If so, how is the test done (anonymous or confidential)? How are results verified and recorded? How much does the test cost? Is pre- and posttest counseling offered?

## Alternative to "Visit or Call a Clinic" Homework

### NOTE TO THE TEACHER

In some communities, individual visits to a clinic may be impractical because of distance, the availability of only one small clinic, or student concerns about confidentiality. Since person-to-person contact with health care providers is important to increasing use of protection, some teachers may not be satisfied with having the majority of students telephoning the clinic. In addition, clinics may not want to receive a lot of calls from one class. In either or any case, two other alternatives are suggested. When alternative activities are used, students can still complete both pages of the homework.

1. *Speakers.* Invite someone from a family planning clinic to speak to the class. Most family planning offices (public hospitals, public health clinics and walk-in comprehensive care centers) are able to provide a speaker who will describe what happens at a clinic and present a film or lecture about family planning methods and HIV and other STD prevention. Such a visitor would help students think of the family planning clinic as more "teen friendly." If there is no film, encourage the speaker to do a role play (perhaps with your assistance).

2. *Field Trips.* Some clinics are willing to host students in small groups. This would almost certainly require that the class be split into smaller groups. The field trips would take some planning, but would ensure that students actually visited a clinic—another important aspect of increasing use of protection. Clinic staff may be willing to lead the field trip.

NOTE TO THE TEACHER

> Be sure to clarify the answers to likely questions during your pre-lesson contacts with clinics.

The timing of this lesson may vary significantly depending on which approach you take to the **Visit or Call a Clinic** assignment. There may be time to complete **How Will You Avoid Pregnancy?** (Worksheet 8.3) in class. If not, do not send it home as homework. Students should have a chance to focus on **Visit or Call a Clinic**.

## How Will You Avoid Pregnancy?

Pass out **How Will You Avoid Pregnancy?** (Worksheet 8.3). Tell students this worksheet gives them a chance to review and personalize the abstinence and protection information they have learned to date. These worksheets are for students to use for their own information and not for class discussion or teacher review. Explain that this worksheet focuses only on birth control. To prevent infection from HIV or other STD, other methods may be required.

## How Is HIV Infection Prevented?

Pass out **How Is HIV Infection Prevented?** (Handout 8.4). Tell students this handout provides information on a number of ways to protect yourself from HIV or lower your risk of HIV infection. Outside of class they can individually assess how well they are protecting themselves from HIV infection.

## Lesson Summary

Remind students that knowing where to go, how to get there and whom to talk to about protection is an important aspect of responsible sexual behavior. Explain that you realize they may not need this information just yet, but they will most likely need this information at some point in their lives. And they may know someone who needs the information now. A person-to-person visit with a health care provider is the best way to find information so students can use it as soon as they are ready to have sex, not after.

Name ____________________

# Visit or Call a Clinic

1. Name of clinic ____________________

2. Address and phone number of clinic ____________________
____________________

3. Clinic is open from _____ a.m. to _____ p.m. _____ days a week.

4. The following services are available at this clinic:
Birth control _____ Prenatal care _____ STD treatment _____
Pregnancy tests _____ Sterilization _____ Counseling _____
HIV antibody test _____

5. A routine examination or consultation about birth control information costs $ ________.

6. Most states have laws that clinics can't disclose information about clients without written consent, including whether or not clients visit the clinic. This is called "client confidentiality." This clinic's confidentiality policy is as follows:
____________________
____________________
____________________

7. Besides English, the following languages are spoken at this clinic: ____________________
____________________

8. I felt the following level of comfort in this clinic (include such things as decor, friendliness of staff, magazines/pamphlets available in waiting room, etc.):

| 1 | 2 | 3 | 4 |
|---|---|---|---|
| Very comfortable | Fairly comfortable | Somewhat comfortable | Uncomfortable |

9. I would/wouldn't tell a friend to visit this clinic for an examination/information consultation about protection. Write two sentences telling why or why not.
____________________
____________________
____________________
____________________

10. Something I learned at this clinic is ____________________
____________________
____________________

***Reminder: Attach a card or brochure from the clinic.***

Name ______________________________

# The Way to the Clinic

**Bus or Train Route from School to the Clinic***

Which bus do you catch? Number or name of bus ______________________________

Where do you get on the bus? ______________________________

Do you need to transfer? Yes No

What are the transfers? ______________________________

Where do you get off? ______________________________

About how far did you have to walk from the last bus to the clinic?

______________________________

______________________________

**Car, Bike or Walking Route from School to the Clinic***

Describe the route from your house or the school to the clinic. Give all street names and freeway numbers. Try to remember and write down other landmarks (like a fast food restaurant or a park) that cue you when to turn. On the attached sheet of paper or map, I have described the:

___ Car Route

___ Bike Route

___ Walking Route

*You may attach a map and mark the route.

# How Will You Avoid Pregnancy?

*Directions:* This worksheet is for your own use and information. It is not for class discussion and will not be turned in to the teacher.

1. Which method(s) for preventing pregnancy would you like to know more about? __

________________________________________

________________________________________

2. How will you find that out? ____________________________

________________________________________

3. Which method seems most convenient? ________________________

4. Which method has the fewest side effects that worry you? _______________

________________________________________

5. Which methods are effective enough for you? ______________________

________________________________________

6. Which method do you think your boyfriend or girlfriend will be most interested in using? ________________________________

________________________________________

7. Which method would your parent(s) be most likely to approve? _____________

________________________________________

8. Show your conclusions from this self-exam by circling the numbers that show which methods seem best for *you.*

| | Best Choice | OK Choice | Worst Choice |
|---|---|---|---|
| Abstinence | 1 | 2 | 3 |
| Condoms | 1 | 2 | 3 |
| Foam | 1 | 2 | 3 |
| Condoms + Foam | 1 | 2 | 3 |
| Pill | 1 | 2 | 3 |
| Norplant | 1 | 2 | 3 |
| Depo Provera | 1 | 2 | 3 |

# How Is HIV Infection Prevented?

*Directions:* The information below will be discussed in class. For your own use, assess how well you are protecting yourself from HIV infection.

**Effectiveness of Methods for Protection from Pregnancy and/or HIV**

| Method | Protects for Pregnancy & HIV | Protects for Pregnancy Only | Doesn't Protect for Either |
|---|---|---|---|
| Withdrawal | | | X |
| Douching | | | X |
| Hoping | | | X |
| Rhythm | | | X |
| Birth Control Pill | | X | |
| Norplant | | X | |
| Depo Provera | | X | |
| Abstinence | X | | |
| Latex Condom | X | | |
| Contraceptive Foam | | X (Fair) | |

**Protect Yourself**

1. Abstinence (not having sex) is the best way to prevent sexual transmission of HIV.

   If you do have sex:

   - You can engage in sex that does not put you in contact with someone else's blood, semen or vaginal fluids.
   - Use a new latex condom and a water-based lubricant every time you have sex.

2. Abstain from alcohol and other drugs, since they affect your judgment and using them may lead to unsafe sex or injection drug use.

   If you do inject drugs:

   - Never share needles or works.

# CLASS 9

# KNOWING AND TALKING ABOUT PROTECTION: SKILLS INTEGRATION—I

## SYNOPSIS

Class 9 is the first of three lessons that provide students the opportunity to practice the communication skills they have just learned using the information and experiences from earlier lessons on protection, birth control methods and clinic services. Students take a quiz on protection methods, then watch role plays in which friends talk to each other about issues related to sex. A discussion follows about ways to handle similar situations.

## PREPARATION

- Review Appendix C, "How to Use Role Plays."
- For each student, locate **Protection: Myths and Truths** (Worksheet 6.3) with Round 1 previously completed.
- Review **Protection: Myths and Truths** (Teacher Key 9.1).
- Two copies of **An Important Discussion** (Role Play 9.2).
- Two copies of **A Lunchtime Chat** (Role Play 9.3).

# OUTLINE OF ACTIVITIES

| Activity | Time | Materials |
|---|---|---|
| Protection: Myths and Truths, Round 2 | 15 minutes | **Protection: Myths and Truths** (Teacher Key 9.1) |
| Demonstrate and Practice Role Play | 30 minutes | **An Important Discussion** (Role Play 9.2) |
| Demonstrate and Practice Role Play | 30 minutes | **A Lunchtime Chat** (Role Play 9.3) |

# ACTIVITIES

## Protection: Myths and Truths, Round 2

1. Have students return to **Protection: Myths and Truths** (Worksheet 6.3) and complete the worksheet, making use of the new information they have learned. They should fill in the Round 2 column of the worksheet.

2. After students have completed the worksheet, review each answer using Teacher Key 9.1. Clarify answers as necessary. Ask students if they scored better on the Round 2 column. Discuss as time allows.

## Demonstrate and Practice Role Play

1. Introduce the friend-to-friend role plays **An Important Discussion** (Role Play 9.2) and **A Lunchtime Chat** (Role Play 9.3). Tell students that many judgments about sexuality and protection are often made by talking with friends and that it's important to talk to friends in a way that protects our decisions. Explain that if they change their minds about a particular decision (give up what they want) just by talking to a friend, they are more likely to give up what they want when they are talking to a boyfriend or girlfriend. On the other hand, if they stick with what they want during talks with friends, they are more likely to be clear and firm when a potentially sexual situation with a boyfriend or girlfriend comes up.

2. Using **An Important Discussion** (Role Play 9.2) and then **A Lunchtime Chat** (Role Play 9.3), demonstrate a discussion between friends with a same-sex student volunteer. After the role plays, ask the class to provide input on other ways to talk about and handle similar situations. To encourage discussion, repeat each line in the role plays and ask for possible responses from the class.

3. Have students divide into groups as usual and role-play. This time, boys will role-play with boys and girls with girls (although the role play can involve a boy and a girl). There is no **Observer Checklist** for these role plays.

4. Ask the class to provide examples of other situations that arise when friends talk to each other about things related to sex. Extract useful responses.

NOTE TO THE TEACHER

If time permits, and **How Will You Avoid Pregnancy?** (Worksheet 8.3) was not completed earlier, have students complete it now.

# Protection: Myths and Truths

1. *The best way to use a condom is to pull it on tight.*

   **MYTH**. The best way is to leave some space at the tip to catch the semen. If the condom has a reservoir tip, you can pull it on tighter.

2. *Teenagers can obtain birth control pills from family planning clinics and doctors without permission from a parent.*

   **TRUTH**. You do not need a parent's permission to get birth control at a clinic. No one needs to know that you are going to a clinic.

3. *Girls can get pregnant if the penis doesn't actually enter the vagina.*

   **TRUTH**. Sperm deposited on the outside of the vagina can make it into the vagina and on up into the fallopian tubes. Sperm can even get through underwear.

4. *Using a latex condom correctly every time you have sexual intercourse is very effective in preventing HIV infection.*

   **TRUTH.** Next to abstinence, this is the most effective protection against HIV infection.

5. *Girls can get pregnant if they have sex during their periods.*

   **TRUTH**. Girls can get pregnant at any time during their cycles, especially if they have short or irregular cycles.

6. *Birth control pills used alone are effective in preventing sexually transmitted disease (STD).*

   **MYTH.** Birth control pills do not prevent STD.

7. *Douching after sex will wash out the sperm and protect against pregnancy and STD.*

   **MYTH**. A girl can't douche fast enough to catch the sperm, and douching may even help the sperm reach the tubes faster. Douching does not kill or wash out the microorganisms that cause STD.

8. *A woman is protected from pregnancy the day she begins taking the pill.*

   **MYTH**. Most physicians recommend that women abstain or use an additional method of birth control for the cycle after she begins using the pill. After this initial period, the woman is protected every day, including during her period.

9. *Abstinence is the most effective method of avoiding HIV infection.*

**TRUTH.** Not having sexual intercourse is the safest, simplest, most effective way to avoid pregnancy, HIV and other STD.

10. *Condoms are effective because they don't break easily and they don't leak.*

**TRUTH**. Condoms are very effective, depending on how carefully they are used. They are also good protection against sexually transmitted disease (STD), including HIV. Condoms are inspected before being marketed, and safety regulations require that condoms be able to hold a large amount of air without breaking. Condoms should not be exposed to heat or Vaseline, as both can cause the rubber to deteriorate which increases chances of breaking.

11. *Sharing needles to inject drugs is one way to get HIV.*

**TRUTH.** Blood with HIV in it may be left in the needle and passed on to the next user.

12. *If a guy pulls his penis out of a girl in time (before he ejaculates), he can be sure to prevent pregnancy.*

**MYTH.** As soon as a male gets an erection, fluid can carry enough sperm into his urethra to escape into the vagina and cause pregnancy, even before ejaculation. Men have no control over the release of this fluid. Withdrawal may, however, offer some protection. It is better than nothing for couples who have unprotected sex.

13. *Pregnant women who are infected with HIV can pass it on to the baby before it is born.*

**TRUTH.** HIV can be passed on to the fetus in the womb, or to the baby during birth or breastfeeding. About one out of every four babies born to HIV-infected mothers will develop HIV.

# An Important Discussion

*Setting the stage:*

Two friends are leaving campus at the end of the day, discussing their feelings about using condoms.

**Friend:** You know, I just hate using condoms!

**You:** Shhh. People can hear us.

**Friend:** Do you want me to use the word "rubber" instead?

**You:** You can use the word "condom." I just get embarrassed talking about those things...I don't like them either.

**Friend:** I just don't like to stop what's going on. You lose something. And...I like the way it feels without it. It feels more...well, natural.

**You:** Yeah, I know what you mean. But you know what we've learned in class. That if you're having sex, condoms and foam are the best protection against pregnancy and STD.

**Friend:** I guess you're right. I'll just have to change my attitude and be sure we use them. My life's pretty good now. I want to keep it that way.

**You:** That's how I feel. This way, we can do everything we're planning to do in high school and then afterward.

# A Lunchtime Chat

*Setting the stage:*

You are talking to a friend at lunch. You tell your friend that you and your boyfriend or girlfriend are thinking about going to a family planning clinic and getting the pill. Your friend doesn't think the pill is a good method and speaks first.

**Friend**: Watch out, the pill might make you (your girlfriend) gain weight.

**You**:

**Friend**: But doesn't the pill give you (your girlfriend) cancer?

**You**:

**Friend**: Anyway, you'll have to tell your (her) mother because you probably need her permission to get the pill.

**You**:

**Friend:** Isn't it really expensive to take the pill?

**You**:

**Friend**: I know I'd never remember to take a pill every day.

**You**:

**Friend**: What will you use to prevent STD? The pill won't protect you against getting HIV infection!

**You**:

# CLASS 10

## SKILLS INTEGRATION—II

### SYNOPSIS

Lesson 10 provides students with further opportunities to practice the skills they are learning to help them say no and to make decisions about protection. In addition to partially scripted role plays, students are presented with "situations" in which they must decide as a group how to handle difficult predicaments.

### PREPARATION

- Review Appendix C, "How to Use Role Plays."
- Four copies each of **Situation A** and **B** (Group Handout 10.1 and 10.2).
- Classroom set of **Two Hours to Kill** (Role Play 10.3) and **A Small Party** (Role Play 10.4).
- Copy classroom set of **Observer Checklist** (Form 10.5).
- *Optional:* Have ready *Refusals* and *Delaying Tactics* Posters and *Role Play Cards* from *Reducing the Risk Supplementary Kit.*

# OUTLINE OF ACTIVITIES

| Activity | Time | Materials |
|---|---|---|
| Review Refusals | 5–10 minutes | *Refusals* and *Delaying Tactics* Posters *(optional)* |
| Generating Alternatives | 15–25 minutes | **Situation A** (Group Handout 10.1) **Situation B** (Group Handout 10.2) |
| Role-Play in Small Groups | 15–25 minutes | **Two Hours to Kill** (Role Play 10.3) **A Small Party** (Role Play 10.4) **Observer Checklist** (Form 10.5) *Refusals* and *Delaying Tactics* Posters and *Role Play Cards (optional)* |

# ACTIVITIES

## Review Refusals

Have students recall behaviors of effective refusals—that is (1) use the word no, (2) repeat no, (3) suggest an alternative, (4) use body language to send a nonverbal no, and (5) build the relationship.

*Optional:* Review the skills students have learned, using the *Refusals* and *Delaying Tactics* Posters from the Supplementary Kit.

## Generating Alternatives

1. Tell students this activity will have them consider an important part of refusals—suggesting an alternative.

2. Divide class into four mixed-sex groups. Give **Situations A** and **B** (Group Handouts 10.1 and 10.2) to each group. Give one person in each group the situation sheet and ask him or her to record the alternatives the group discusses.

3. Give groups a couple of minutes to read the situations and then list as many alternatives as they can for each. Explain that the goal is to think of as many options as they can and to look at the situation from as many points of view as possible.

4. Have a volunteer from each group present their suggestions regarding **Situation A** to the class. Reinforce the number of options provided by the class—having a lot of options in mind will help them find ways to live up to their decisions not to have unprotected sex. If one idea doesn't work, they can always try another. "Withdrawal" and "finding something similar to a rubber around the house" should, of course, be discouraged. Being able to think imaginatively is a step toward avoiding confrontations and situations that ruin relationships and can lead to pregnancy or infection with HIV or another STD.

## Role-Play in Small Groups

1. Suggest to students that the alternatives they have just suggested could be used in the next role plays, **Two Hours to Kill** (Role Play 10.3) and **A Small Party** (Role Play 10.4).

2. Have the groups stay together and hand out both role plays. Again, instruct students to alternate the roles in the unscripted parts. Make sure each student has the chance to be in the unscripted role. Have students use the **Observer Checklist** (Form 10.5). Walk around and facilitate student-to-student feedback.

   *Optional:* Pass out a set of *Role Play Cards* to each group. Ask each member to take one card. Review each role with the whole group. Write key words on the board:

   - Student Role Player #1: Read lines.
   - Student Role Player #2: Respond to lines.
   - Student Observer #1: Set the stage for the role play, and use **Observer Checklist** (Form 10.5).
   - Student Observer #2: Use **Observer Checklist** (Form 10.5) and lead small group discussion using the guidelines on the back of the card.

# Situation A

Taylor and Bobby have gone out for a long time but have never had sex. One day they go to Bobby's sister's apartment. She is in the bedroom with her boyfriend. In the living room, Taylor and Bobby start to kiss and warm up to each other.

What can Taylor or Bobby do to avoid sex or unprotected sex?

*List alternative actions below:*

# Situation B

Tony and Dylan have been to a party and then go to Tony's home to be alone. They start to kiss and undress each other. Dylan reaches into his jacket pocket, and realizes that he doesn't have the condom he planned to use. He says, "I think somebody stole the rubber I had."

What can Tony and Dylan do to avoid unprotected sex?

*List alternative actions below:*

# Two Hours to Kill

*Setting the stage:*

You are at your boyfriend's (girlfriend's) house after school. You aren't ready to have sex and you've said so. You know no one will be home for two hours. You are kissing and touching and your boyfriend (girlfriend) lets you know he (she) wants to make love. You do not want to make love.

**Person 1:** It's OK to have sex when you love each other.

**Person 2:**

**Person 1:** We don't get many chances to be alone.

**Person 2:**

**Person 1:** You're not worried about getting pregnant or infected, are you?

**Person 2:**

**Person 1:** OK then, we'll use a condom.

**Person 2:**

**Person 1:** I just feel so close to you. That's why I want to have sex.

**Person 2:**

**Person 1:** If you loved me as much as I love you, you'd do it.

**Person 2:**

**Person 1:**

**Person 2:**

# A Small Party

*Setting the stage:*

You've been going out with someone for six months and care for this person very much. There's going to be a small party at a good friend's house and the two of you can be alone. Your partner asks you to get some protection before the party. You're not ready to have sex. Your partner says:

**Partner 1:** I guess you don't really care about me.

**Partner 2:**

**Partner 1:** I feel like a fool asking you. I never thought you'd act like this.

**Partner 2:**

**Partner 1:** Are you starting to see someone else?

**Partner 2:**

**Partner 1:** Well, I thought you'd really want to do it.

**Partner 2:**

**Partner 1:** What if I got the protection?

**Partner 2:**

**Partner 1:** This takes the fun out of going to the party.

**Partner 2:**

**Partner 1:** I guess it's not so important, right now.

**Partner 2:**

Name: ______________________ Date: ______________________

# Observer Checklist

ROLE PLAY #

| REFUSALS | 1 | 2 | 3 | 4 | 5 | 6 |
|---|---|---|---|---|---|---|
| Said "NO" | | | | | | |
| Body Language Said "NO" | | | | | | |
| Repeated Refusal | | | | | | |
| Suggested Alternative | | | | | | |
| Built the Relationship | | | | | | |
| DELAYING TACTICS | | | | | | |
| Used Delay Statement | | | | | | |
| Used Delay Action | | | | | | |
| Created Space | | | | | | |
| Ended the Situation Quickly | | | | | | |
| Built the Relationship | | | | | | |

# CLASS 11

## SKILLS INTEGRATION—III

### SYNOPSIS

Class 11 provides continued opportunities for students to practice handling situations that might otherwise lead to unprotected sex.

### PREPARATION

- Review Appendix C, "How to Use Role Plays."
- For each student, copy **My Kid Sister** (Worksheet 11.1).
- For each student, copy **Time for a Condom** (Role Play 11.2).
- For each student, copy **Observer Checklist** (Form 11.3).
- *Optional:* Have ready *Role Play Cards* from *Reducing the Risk Supplementary Kit.*

### OUTLINE OF ACTIVITIES

| Activity | Time | Materials |
|---|---|---|
| My Kid Sister | 10–25 minutes | **My Kid Sister** (Worksheet 11.1) |
| Role-Play in Small Groups | 20–30 minutes | **Time for a Condom** (Role Play 11.2) **Observer Checklist** (Form 11.3) *Role Play Cards (optional)* |

# ACTIVITIES

## My Kid Sister

Hand out **My Kid Sister** (Worksheet 11.1). Tell students to complete the form according to the directions on the worksheet. Remind them of communication skills they might use (relationship building, suggesting an alternative, and helping her delay). Allow approximately ten minutes for students to complete the worksheet. When they are finished, discuss:

a. best reasons not to have sex

b. reasons to have sex

c. good ways to encourage kids not to have sex

## Role-Play in Small Groups

As before, divide students into groups and have students role-play **Time for a Condom** (Role Play 11.2). This is an equal opportunity role play and males or females can play either part. Again, instruct students to alternate roles in the unscripted part. Make sure each student has the chance to be in the unscripted role. Have students use the **Observer Checklist** (Form 11.3). Walk around and facilitate student-to-student feedback. *This time,* tell students that they don't have to use the scripts. After reading the situation, they can create their own lines if they wish.

*Optional:* Pass out a set of *Role Play Cards* to each group. Ask each member to take one card. Review each role with the whole group. Write key words on the board:

- Student Role Player #1: Read lines.
- Student Role Player #2: Respond to lines.
- Student Observer #1: Set the stage for the role play, and use **Observer Checklist** (Form 11.3).
- Student Observer #2: Use **Observer Checklist** (Form 11.3) and lead small group discussion using the guidelines on the back of the card.

# My Kid Sister

*Directions:* Imagine that you have a younger sister who is 12 years old. She tells you she wants to have sex with her boyfriend. You don't think she should have sex yet. Write what you would say to her.

**Sister**: He really wants me to and I love him.

**You**:

**Sister**: He's the cutest boy in school.

**You**:

**Sister**: I'm going to do it someday, anyway. What's wrong with now?

**You**:

**Sister**: He said he'd use a condom.

**You**:

**Sister**: We really love each other.

**You**:

**Sister**: If I lose him, I'll just die.

**You**:

# Time for a Condom

*Setting the stage:*

You and your boyfriend (girlfriend) have had sex without using protection. You just found out a close friend is pregnant and you don't want it to happen to you. You want to talk about using a condom, but you're nervous so you've put it off. Now you're alone together in a RED ALERT situation. You stop and say you want to talk.

**Person 1:**

**Person 2:** Now? What do you want to talk about at a time like this?

**Person 1:**

**Person 2:** We've done it before and you're (I'm) not pregnant.

**Person 1:**

**Person 2:** Let's talk about it next time, OK? Don't spoil the mood.

**Person 1:**

**Person 2:** I don't want to use protection. I don't think it would feel right.

**Person 1:**

**Person 2:** Nothing's going to happen. My sister has sex without protection. She's not pregnant, and she doesn't have HIV either.

**Person 1:**

**Person 2:** Other couples do it without protection.

**Person 1:**

**Person 2:** I just think it will take away half the fun.

**Person 1:**

**Person 2:** Sounds like you're really serious. I guess a condom is easy to get.

**Person 1:**

**Person 2:**

Name: ____________________ Date: ____________________

# Observer Checklist

ROLE PLAY #

| REFUSALS | 1 | 2 | 3 | 4 | 5 | 6 |
|---|---|---|---|---|---|---|
| Said "NO" | | | | | | |
| Body Language Said "NO" | | | | | | |
| Repeated Refusal | | | | | | |
| Suggested Alternative | | | | | | |
| Built the Relationship | | | | | | |
| DELAYING TACTICS | | | | | | |
| Used Delay Statement | | | | | | |
| Used Delay Action | | | | | | |
| Created Space | | | | | | |
| Ended the Situation Quickly | | | | | | |
| Built the Relationship | | | | | | |

# CLASS 12

# PREVENTING HIV AND OTHER STD

## SYNOPSIS

Accurate information about sexually transmitted disease, particularly how to prevent transmission, is the foundation for reducing risk behaviors. To help students understand the commonalities of STD, including HIV, and how to protect themselves from sexually transmitted disease, they work in small groups to explore information about transmission and prevention of five specific STDs. Groups compare the ways these STDs are transmitted, how they are prevented, how to get treatment, and then make some conclusions about sexually transmitted disease in general, including HIV.

## PREPARATION

- Obtain a classroom set of *STD Facts* and *HIV Facts* (pamphlets available from ETR Associates) or other pamphlets on STD from a local resource.
- Review **Teacher Background Information About HIV** (Teacher Reference 12.1).
- Copy a classroom set of **How HIV Would Change My Life** (Homework 12.2).

# OUTLINE OF ACTIVITIES

| Activity | Time | Materials |
|---|---|---|
| Facts About STD Including HIV | 40–80 minutes (up to two classes) | Classroom set of *STD Facts* and *HIV Facts* or other pamphlets **Teacher Background Information About HIV** (Teacher Reference 12.1) |
| Assign Homework | 5 minutes | **How HIV Would Change My Life** (Homework 12.2) |

# ACTIVITIES

## Facts About STD, Including HIV

1. Tell students that sexually transmitted disease (STD) is not a single disease but actually a group of communicable diseases that are spread through intimate (usually sexual) contact. Another name for STD is "venereal disease," which, historically, came from the name Venus, the goddess of love. STD is the new terminology and can be used interchangeably with VD when referring to diseases that are transmitted by intimate sexual contact. **About one in eight teenagers currently has an STD.**

2. Write the names of five common STDs across the top of the board: genital warts, gonorrhea, herpes, chlamydia and HIV. Divide the class into five groups. Provide each student with pamphlet(s) on STD. Ask each group to pick one of these five STDs to study. On the board, cross out each STD as it is picked so it will be used only *once*. Instruct each group to identify the following five characteristics about the STD they have chosen and record them on paper.
   a. how I could get it
   b. how I can prevent it
   c. how I would know I have it (symptoms)
   d. how I would get treatment
   e. how it would change my life

NOTE TO THE TEACHER

> One option is to give each group a piece of butcher paper with the name of an STD at the top. Have them write in large letters. Then post all papers side by side.

3. Give groups about ten minutes to research the STD. Then, ask each group to provide a summary statement for each of the five points on each STD.

4. After all groups have reported, pull five summary statements that are true about all these STDs on each point. *For example:*
   a. You can get STD, including HIV, from intimate sexual contact with someone who has the disease.
   b. You can prevent STD, including HIV, by abstaining; by having a lifelong, monogamous sexual relationship with a mutually faithful, uninfected partner; or by reducing the risk by using a latex condom.
   c. STD, including HIV, can damage an unborn baby, make you sterile, and weaken your general health.
   d. Having an STD has a social stigma and is embarrassing.
   e. You should go to a clinic or see a physician if you see any symptoms.
   f. At first, a person with an STD will look and feel healthy but can still transmit the disease to others.

5. Ask how HIV differs from the other STDs.
   a. You get HIV infection from blood, semen and vaginal secretions.
   b. HIV is significantly more lethal than the other STDs. For adults, the average length of time between becoming HIV-infected and being diagnosed with AIDS can be as long as ten years. There are no medically documented cases of people who have recovered from HIV.
   c. HIV receives much more attention from the press.
   d. People are more afraid of HIV than of other STD.
   e. Many heterosexuals do not consider themselves to be at risk for HIV.
   f. HIV may be transmitted by sharing injection needles.

## Assign Homework

1. Hand out the homework **How HIV Would Change My Life** (Homework 12.2).

2. Collect homework in another class and discuss as time permits.

# Teacher Background Information About HIV

This section provides the teacher with information about HIV.

## I. What Is HIV?

HIV (human immunodeficiency virus) is the virus that causes AIDS (Acquired Immune Deficiency Syndrome).

People who have HIV in their bodies are said to have HIV infection or be HIV-positive. HIV damages the body's immune system. The immune system protects the body from disease. HIV infection is a disease with many stages. An HIV-positive person can range from being healthy to being very sick. People can have HIV for years without getting sick. They may look and feel healthy. They may not even know they are infected.

## II. What Is AIDS?

AIDS is the stage when an HIV-positive person's immune system gets very weak. When this happens, other diseases and infections can enter the body.

The diagnosis of AIDS is made when a person's T-cell count drops below 200 or when a person develops one or more of several specific conditions that indicate critical impairment of the immune system. These include *Pneumocystis carinii* pneumonia (PCP), Kaposi's sarcoma (KS), pulmonary tuberculosis (TB), recurrent pneumonia and, in women, invasive cervical cancer.

## III. How Do People Get Infected with HIV? (How Is HIV Transmitted?)

Anyone can become infected with HIV, regardless of age, sex, race, sexual orientation, or anything else. HIV is transmitted through blood, semen and vaginal secretions. It is most commonly transmitted from an infected person to an uninfected person in the following ways:

- Through anal, vaginal or oral intercourse. HIV is in the blood, semen and vaginal fluids of someone with HIV. Anyone who has sex (heterosexual or gay/lesbian) with someone who has HIV can get HIV.
- By sharing needles used for injection drug use or injecting vitamins or steroids. Blood with HIV in it may be left in the needle or syringe and passed on to the next user. (There is also a theoretical risk from sharing needles for tattooing or piercing, although there are no documented cases of HIV transmission by this method.)
- From mother to child either before or during birth. There are also a few known cases in which HIV has been passed from mother to child through breast milk.

The virus can also be transmitted by receiving blood transfusions, blood components, tissues or organs from donors infected with the virus. Transmission in this manner is very rare (about one in 40,000 persons) since 1985, when testing for HIV was implemented.

## IV. How HIV Is Not Transmitted

HIV is **not** transmitted by normal day-to-day contact between people (at home, school or work, or elsewhere in the community), nor is it transmitted through the air.

HIV is not transmitted in the following ways:

- touching, coughing, sneezing or dry kissing
- contact with toilet seats, eating utensils, water fountains or telephones
- using facilities such as swimming pools, restrooms or gymnasiums
- being close to other people in a classroom, restaurant, a crowded bus or other facility
- mosquitoes or other biting insects
- donating blood (all equipment is sterile)
- tears or saliva

## V. Who Is at Risk?

It is not who you are but what you do that puts you at risk. Anyone who has sex or shares needles with an HIV-infected person can become HIV-infected.

You are at risk for HIV infection if:

- You are (or have ever been) a sex partner (heterosexual or gay/lesbian) of someone who is HIV-positive or someone at risk for HIV infection.
- You have shared needles to inject drugs, steroids or vitamins, or for tattooing or piercing.
- You have ever had sex (heterosexual or gay/lesbian) with an injection drug user.
- You have ever had sex with a man or woman who has had sex with another person.
- You have ever had sex with someone with hemophilia.
- You have ever had sex with someone who had a blood transfusion before 1985.
- You have hemophilia or received a blood transfusion before 1985.
- You have ever been sexually assaulted.
- You have ever had a sexually transmitted disease (STD).
- Babies born to women with HIV are also at risk.

## VI. How Can People Eliminate or Reduce the Risk of Becoming HIV-Infected?

*Risk elimination:*

- Do not engage in sexual intercourse.
- Do not use injection drugs.
- If sexually active, remain in a relationship with only one partner who is not infected, not using injection drugs, not sharing needles or syringes, and not having sexual intercourse with other partners.

*Risk reduction:*

- Openly discuss with a partner the possibility of HIV infection. Listen for clues of past or present risk behaviors.
- Avoid having more than one sex partner. The more sex partners a person has, the greater the chance of contracting HIV or another STD.
- Avoid contact with a partner's blood, semen or vaginal secretions.
- Properly use latex condoms (not lambskin or natural membrane) during each instance of sexual intercourse.
- If unwilling to seek treatment for injection drug use, do not share needles. If needles are shared, clean them three times with water, three times with full-strength bleach and three times again with water before each use.
- Do not share needles or other sharp piercing instruments for tattooing, piercing or acupuncture unless they are sterilized.
- Do not use alcohol, marijuana or other drugs that impair judgment and weaken the immune system.

## VII. What Is the HIV Test?

The HIV tests currently being used can indicate whether a person has been infected with HIV by detecting the antibodies the human body makes as a result of such infection. These tests do not show whether a person has or will develop AIDS.

Due to the possibility of occasional false positive and false negative results, a series of tests are performed on the same blood sample. An initial test is generally performed twice. If either test is positive, a different confirmatory test is used to check the results. A confirmed positive test means antibodies to HIV are present. The tested individual is then known to have been infected with HIV, and is presumed to be able to infect other people.

If the two initial tests are negative, no confirmatory test is performed and the test is reported as negative. This means no antibodies to HIV were detected, and most likely the person tested is not infected. However, a person recently exposed and infected (generally within six months prior to testing), may not yet have developed antibodies that can be detected by the test. If an individual has tested negative but has had some HIV-related risk within the past six months, it would be best to be tested again after the six-month period has passed to be confident of the results. The sooner people are tested, the sooner those who are HIV-positive can begin health practices and treatment that can slow the progress of the disease and keep them healthy.

Tests are available at public health clinics, hospitals, doctors' offices and other locations. When selecting a testing site, a person may wish to find out whether the test is anonymous or confidential, how results are verified and recorded, and if counseling is part of the procedure.

## VIII. What Are the Symptoms of HIV Infection?

Many of the symptoms of HIV infection are also symptoms of minor illnesses or infections. But with HIV the symptoms either don't go away or keep coming back. Many people with HIV do not have any symptoms for a long time. See a doctor if any of these symptoms persist and you have had any known HIV risk:

- unexplained weight loss greater than ten pounds
- recurring fever and/or drenching night sweats
- unexplained persistent tiredness
- chronic diarrhea
- swollen glands, usually in the neck, armpits or groin
- unexplained persistent dry cough
- white spots or unusual sores on the tongue or mouth

Women with yeast infections that keep coming back, pelvic inflammatory disease (PID), genital warts, ovarian or cervical disease, or abnormal Pap smears should ask about HIV testing.

## IX. How Long Can a Person Be Infected with HIV Before Being Diagnosed with AIDS?

The length of time between becoming HIV-infected and being diagnosed with AIDS, sometimes called the "incubation period" for AIDS, varies from person to person. In rare cases, it may be as little as a few weeks or months. Some people have had HIV infection for 12 years or longer and still do not have an AIDS diagnosis. The average length of time between being infected with HIV and being diagnosed with AIDS is approximately eight to ten years.

## X. Will Everyone with HIV Die?

For most people with HIV, the condition has been progressive and deteriorative—over time people get sicker, and the immune system becomes increasingly impaired. There are no medically documented cases of people who have recovered from HIV. However, there are many people living with HIV today who have done well for years.

## XI. Is There a Vaccine, Cure or Treatment?

At the present time, prevention is the only "vaccine" for HIV. There is no cure for HIV, and a true cure is certainly many years away, if it is even possible. A number of medications have been developed which slow progression of HIV. There are also treatments that can help prevent some of the common illnesses that develop in people with HIV. Some people with HIV also use non-Western and nonmedical approaches to address their infection. Acupuncture, herbal and Chinese medicine, homeopathy, visualization, vitamins and support groups have all been used, sometimes along with traditional Western medicine.

# How HIV Would Change My Life

1. If I had HIV, I would have to make the following changes in the way I act with my romantic partners:

   A. ______

   B. ______

   C. ______

2. If I had HIV, it would harm me in these ways:

   A. ______

   B. ______

   C. ______

3. The most difficult thing for me about being HIV-positive would be:

   A. ______

   B. ______

   C. ______

4. If I had HIV, my life would change in the following ways:

   A. ______

   B. ______

   C. ______

# CLASS 13

## HIV RISK BEHAVIORS

### SYNOPSIS

The purpose of this activity is to help students apply their knowledge about HIV transmission and identify which behaviors put them at greatest risk for exposure to HIV. Participants place behaviors on a continuum of risk, from no risk to risky, and discuss why some behaviors are more risky than others.

Adolescents need help with understanding that there are no second chances when it comes to HIV infection.

Because symptoms of HIV infection often do not develop for many years, adolescents rarely seek testing for the virus. The lack of data about HIV infection rates is also likely to contribute to teens' views of themselves as having little risk. Students need to know that there is a very long incubation period between HIV infection and a diagnosis of AIDS. About 20 percent of all diagnosed AIDS cases in the United States are people between the ages of 20 and 29. Most were probably infected as teens.

Some adolescents fail to recognize their risk for HIV exposure when they decide to have sex with a steady boyfriend or girlfriend. They believe they are engaging in low-risk behavior because of information that having sex with one long-term partner is the next best approach after abstinence. To adolescents, a steady relationship of six months or even less may qualify as long-term. Unfortunately, a series of such relationships does little to protect anyone from contracting HIV.

Many adolescents do not understand the potential impact of drug or alcohol use on their behavior and fail to recognize such use as a risk factor for HIV transmission.

## PREPARATION

- Draw a traffic light on each of three 5" × 7" index cards. Make one light red, another green and the third yellow. Tape the traffic lights along the wall to create a risk continuum from green to red OR have ready *Traffic Light Cards* from *Reducing the Risk Supplementary Kit (optional).*
- Have one package each of white, blue and pink 3" × 5" index cards. Select behaviors from **Risk Behaviors** (Teacher Reference 13.1.) If the behavior is associated with sexual activity, write it on a white index card. If it is associated with use of needles, write it on a blue card. If it is associated with another mode of transmission, write it on a pink card OR have ready *Risk Behavior Cards* from *Reducing the Risk Supplementary Kit.* You may want to prepare rolled pieces of tape to stick on the back of the cards to facilitate their placement on the wall.
- For each student, make a copy of **Risk Behaviors Answer Sheet** (Handout 13.2).

## OUTLINE OF ACTIVITIES

| Activity | Time | Materials |
|---|---|---|
| Risk Continuum | 25 minutes | **Risk Behaviors** (Teacher Reference 13.1) *Traffic Light Cards* and *Risk Behavior Cards (optional)* |
| Personal Risks | 5 minutes | **Risk Behaviors Answer Sheet** (Handout 13.2) |
| Lesson Summary | 5 minutes | None |

## ACTIVITIES

### Risk Continuum

1. Explain to students that the three traffic lights on the cards taped to the wall represent points along a risk continuum:
   - Red is risky.
   - Yellow is uncertain.
   - Green is virtually no risk.

   Ask students to indicate the level of risk for HIV transmission associated with various behaviors (from Teacher Reference 13.1).

For example:

"Using the same condom twice" would go under the red light, "breastfeeding by an infected mother" would go under the yellow light and "dry kissing" would go under the green light.

2. Organize students into groups of five to seven. Pass out cards with behaviors written on them or the *Risk Behavior Cards.* Give each student at least one card. Explain the color coding of the cards.

3. Ask students to decide within their groups the level of risk of the behaviors on their cards. Encourage groups to come to consensus about where each card belongs on the continuum. Ask students to tape their cards along the wall on the risk continuum.

## NOTE TO THE TEACHER

- Sometimes students will want to know the exact placement of a behavior by its "percentage of risk." Such absolute levels of risk are unknown. However, we do know that some behaviors put us at more risk than others. The point of this activity is to develop skills in evaluating *relative* risk.
- It is important to review the list of behaviors and add or delete any as appropriate for your classroom. An alternative to using a predeveloped list is to ask students to generate their own list of behaviors (after the basic facts are covered).
- Be sure not to leave a card incorrectly placed along the continuum, as visual learners may memorize incorrect placement.
- Heated discussion may emerge about the proper placement of a behavior along the risk continuum. Stress that any behavior not placed under the green light puts us at risk of HIV infection. End any discussion that becomes nonproductive.
- When the students are evaluating a behavior, they may ask you whether the sex partner is infected with HIV. Say that you do not know.

4. When all cards have been placed along the wall, review each behavior and its place along the continuum. Ask if any cards should be moved, discuss why, and do so, if appropriate. Ask for class consensus on where each card belongs. Remind students that the purpose of this activity is to identify the relative risk of behaviors, *not* to judge those who placed the cards.

5. Once the whole class agrees about where each card should be placed along the continuum, ask students to look at the behaviors and privately consider whether they are doing any of these things.

6. Distribute the **Risk Behaviors Answer Sheet** (Handout 13.2). Explain that the answers are based on the latest scientific data. There may be different interpretations of what those behaviors imply, and discussion in groups may have led to a different rating. This is fine, as long as there is an accurate link between a clearly understood behavior and its relative risk. It is easier to identify those behaviors that are clearly safe (green) than to place other behaviors on the continuum from possibly unsafe (yellow) to unsafe (red).

   Emphasize that there is no way to know a person's risk status. Thus, regardless of how well you know your partner, behaviors such as unprotected intercourse must be considered high risk.

## Lesson Summary

Remind students that, as was discussed in the previous lesson, it is not who you are but what you do that puts you at risk.

Stress that anyone who has sex or shares needles with an HIV-infected person can get HIV. Therefore, in order to eliminate their risk of getting HIV, they must not engage in sexual intercourse and must not use injection drugs. People who are sexually active must remain in a lifetime relationship with only one partner who is not infected, not using injection drugs, not sharing needles or syringes, and not having sexual intercourse with other people, or must use latex condoms correctly during each instance of sexual intercourse to protect themselves from HIV.

# HIV Risk Behaviors

**Associated with sexual activity**

Massage
French kissing
Mutual masturbation
Unprotected oral sex
Dry kissing
Abstaining from sex
Unprotected vaginal sex
Fantasizing
Using latex condoms correctly every time
Anal sex
Masturbation
Hugging
Using the same condom twice
Maintaining a lifetime, mutually monogamous relationship with an uninfected partner who does not use injection drugs
Intercourse using an oil-based lubricant and condom

**Associated with use of needles**

Sharing needles for injecting drugs, steroids or vitamins
Reusing a needle that has been cleaned with bleach
Reusing a needle that has been cleaned with water
Sharing needles for tattooing or piercing

**Associated with other modes of transmission**

Receiving a blood transfusion today
Donating blood
Cleaning spilled blood without wearing gloves
Breastfeeding by an infected mother

Adapted with permission from *Training Educators in HIV Prevention* by J. L. Collins and P. O. Britton. 1990. Santa Cruz, CA: ETR Associates.

# HIV Risk Behaviors Answer Sheet

**No Risk**

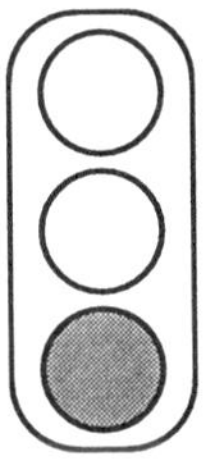

**Some Risk**

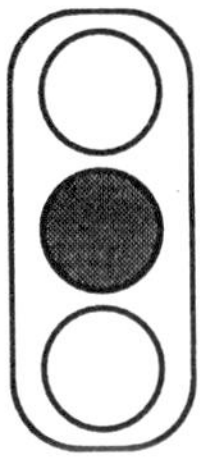

**Risky**

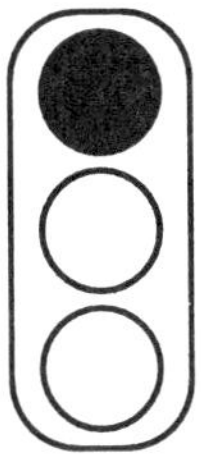

Massage

Receiving a blood transfusion today >>

Dry kissing

Abstaining from sex

Fantasizing

Masturbation

Hugging

Donating blood

Maintaining a lifetime, mutually monogamous relationship with an uninfected partner who does not use injection drugs

French kissing

Properly using condoms with nonoxynol-9 or other spermicide

Mutual masturbation

<< Reusing a needle that has been cleaned with bleach

<< Breast-feeding by an infected mother

Unprotected oral sex >>

Unprotected vaginal sex

Intercourse using an oil-based lubricant and condom

Using the same condom twice

Anal sex

Sharing needles for anything, including injecting drugs, ear piercing, tattooing, and injecting steroids or vitamins

Reusing a needle that has been cleaned with water

Cleaning spilled blood without wearing gloves

<< This behavior could move slightly toward the left of the continuum.
>> This behavior could move slightly toward the right of the continuum.

Adapted with permission from *Training Educators in HIV Prevention* by J. L. Collins and P.O. Britton. 1990. Santa Cruz, CA: ETR Associates.

# CLASS 14

# IMPLEMENTING PROTECTION FROM STD AND PREGNANCY

## SYNOPSIS

The purpose of the activities in Class 14 is to help students develop plans for preventing pregnancy and reducing the risk of STD, including HIV, through the use of a condom. In the first activity, students project on a worksheet what they would say and do to take steps toward protection. Then they use their experience in thinking about these plans to create the content in the role-play activity.

## PREPARATION

- Review Appendix C, "How to Use Role Plays."
- For each student, copy **The Steps to Protection** (Worksheet 14.1)

## OUTLINE OF ACTIVITIES

| Activity | Time | Materials |
|---|---|---|
| The Steps to Protection | 10–25 minutes | **The Steps to Protection** (Worksheet 14.1) |
| Role Plays | 15–25 minutes | None |
| Lesson Summary | 5 minutes | None |

## ACTIVITIES

### The Steps to Protection

1. Tell students the path to self-protection is not without twists and turns. There are several decisions to make, actions to take and troubles to shake. The following exercise gives students a chance to think through the steps to self-protection and to plan ways to achieve their goal of avoiding (or greatly reducing) the risk of pregnancy and exposure to HIV and other sexually transmitted diseases, by the use of condoms.

   Hand out **The Steps to Protection** (Worksheet 14.1) for students to complete. This worksheet should be done alone since it includes some rather personal decisions that each person must make. The idea is to help students develop plans for using condoms for a time in their lives when they might need it. This worksheet is specific to planning for the use of condoms and foam.

2. When most students have completed the first step ("Talking About a Plan for Protection"), discuss it. Volunteers should share ideas for taking steps for self-protection. See if students have the idea of talking about it ahead of time before going on to the next two steps on the worksheet.

### Role Plays

1. Role plays follow up on the individual plans and the class discussion of **The Steps to Protection** (Worksheet 14.1). Put students into small groups of no more than four. Tell them to develop a role play that addresses one of the three steps of preparation for using condoms. Instruct groups to write a script that describes a discus-

sion that might occur in Step 1 while "Talking About a Plan for Protection" or in Step 3, "Using Protection." Have them write a full script on a separate sheet of paper.

2. When students have had a chance to finish the scripts, have them return to the full group and read their role plays aloud to the rest of the class.

## Lesson Summary

Tell students that many of them plan just what they are going to do and say to get a friend to lend them a special coat or a car, to get someone to go out with them, or to persuade their parent(s) to give money to a great cause like themselves. Remind students that they can also plan every detail of how to protect themselves. Today was just a start.

Tell them that if they go all the way with planning, they won't go all the way into trouble.

NOTE TO THE TEACHER

Remind students that the **Shopping Information Form** (Homework 7.1) and **Visit or Call a Clinic** (Homework 8.1) are due in the next class.

# The Steps to Protection

*Directions:* Picture a time in your life when you would be ready to have sex. It may be now, next year or when you're married. Suppose you are concerned about preventing a pregnancy or preventing STD and want to use a condom and foam. The steps to protection are described. You are to write how you would do it.

*Setting the Stage:*

You and your boyfriend or girlfriend have not had sex before, but you have been going out for a long time and have an anniversary coming up next Saturday night. You think it is about time for sex but you are not exactly sure what the other one thinks. You want to be sure that you are protected from HIV and other sexually transmitted disease, and from pregnancy, by saying no or using a condom and foam. The steps to protection are described. You are to write how you would do it. Section 3 is optional.

## STEP 1: Talking About a Plan for Protection

1. *Talk to your partner about using a condom and foam*

   Where will you talk about it? ____________________

   When will you talk about it? ____________________

   What will you say? ____________________

   ____________________

   What problems might arise in planning for protection? ____________________

   ____________________

   What would you do then? ____________________

   ____________________

**STEP 2: Preparing for Protection**

2. *Get the condoms and foam*

Who will get them? ____________________

When? ____________________

Where? ____________________

What problems might arise in getting them? ____________________

____________________

What would you do then? ____________________

____________________

**STEP 3: Using Protection**

3. *Use the condoms and foam*

Whose job would it be to carry the protection? ____________________

Who would bring out the condoms and foam? ____________________

What would he or she say? ____________________

____________________

____________________

What would be the most romantic way to use the condom and foam? ____________________

____________________

____________________

What might go wrong? ____________________

What would you do to save the evening? ____________________

____________________

# CLASS 15

# STICKING WITH ABSTINENCE AND PROTECTION

## SYNOPSIS

Class 15 provides the important opportunity for students to discuss their experiences with the two homework assignments that require them to find information about protection. Additionally, students discuss and practice the "self-talk" method to help them plan and then stick with the plan to avoid sex or unprotected sex.

## PREPARATION

- For each student, copy **Sticking with Abstinence and Protection** (Worksheet 15.1).

# OUTLINE OF ACTIVITIES

| Activity | Time | Materials |
|---|---|---|
| Review Shopping Information and Visit or Call a Clinic Homework | 10–20 minutes | Completed **Shopping Information Form** (Homework 7.1) and **Visit or Call a Clinic** (Homework 8.1) |
| Sticking with Abstinence and Protection | 20–35 minutes | **Sticking with Abstinence and Protection** (Worksheet 15.1) |

# ACTIVITIES

## Review "Shopping Information" and "Visit or Call a Clinic" Homework

1. Ask students what they learned from the trips to price methods of protection or to the family planning clinic and, especially, ask what helped them to complete the assignment despite possible embarrassment. Discuss the **Shopping Information** homework assigned in Class 7. Include the following questions in your discussion:

   a. What did they learn about types and costs of protection?
      Pull for: (1) It is easily available.
      (2) It is inexpensive.
      (3) It was not too embarrassing to look at.

   b. How did they feel about going into the store and looking at condoms and foam?

   c. What was the worst thing that any of them expected would happen? Did anything like that happen? Did anything good happen?

   d. Find out how many of them would recommend the stores they visited. If a lot would recommend theirs, comment that it seems pretty easy to find a store that sells protection in a friendly way.

   e. Find out the typical hours of operation for these stores. Ask who went to a store that they think stayed open the latest. Ask them where they could go to get protection even later than that.

2. Then proceed to discuss the **Visit or Call a Clinic** homework (first assigned in Class 8). In the discussion, help students to inform each other about:
   a. The names and locations of the clinics they visited.
   b. What they expected the clinic would be like and if it was like that.
   c. Ask if anyone had a bad experience visiting the clinic or has questions about the clinic experience.
   d. Ask if anyone had a good experience and any ideas to share with other people about visiting a clinic.
   e. Ask about the confidentiality policies at the clinics and the importance of these policies. Why are these important? (Pull for the idea that sex and sexuality are private and that people should and do have control over their choices to use birth control from clinics or drugstores.)
   f. Ask what languages were spoken at the clinics. Ask why so many languages were spoken. (Pull for idea that clinics are trying to be sure that everyone feels comfortable and gets all the information they need to prevent unwanted pregnancies and infection with HIV or other STD.)
   g. Ask if anyone found a clinic that is especially easy to get to from their home or high school without a car.

## Sticking with Abstinence and Protection

1. Use the following to introduce "self-talk" to students:

   "By now, I hope you all have the goal to delay sex, or at least to avoid pregnancy, HIV and other sexually transmitted disease. Sometimes people may try to talk us out of sticking to our goals. But at other times we may even talk ourselves out of being abstinent or using birth control. You may have doubts about being able to accomplish your goals. You may wonder if you will know what to do when the time comes to avoid sex or pregnancy. For example, imagine that you wanted to use a condom for the first time. What are some of your doubts or worries that would keep you from trying it out?"

   Give them one idea such as, "It's going to spoil it if we have to stop and put on a condom." Have the class volunteer additional ideas. Generate eight to ten ideas for doubts that might get in the way of using a condom. Write the first four ideas on the board.

Leave space for writing "doubt" and for writing "doubt busters." These are things you can do or say to yourself to make using a condom easier. The last four to six ideas can just be listed. "Doubts" and "doubt busters" might include the following examples:

DOUBT: *I'll look like a beginner if I don't know what to do with the condom.*
DOUBT-BUSTER ACTION: I'll practice putting a condom on my fingers so I'm sure I'll know how.

DOUBT: *It will look as if I planned it if I have the condom ready.*
DOUBT-BUSTER ACTION: I could tell him or her that we could go shopping for it together.

DOUBT: *It won't feel as good if we use a condom.*
DOUBT-BUSTER ACTION: Be sure we don't rush so we can enjoy the whole time together before and after the condom.

DOUBT: *He or she won't keep going out with me if I don't have sex.*
DOUBT-BUSTER ACTION: Think of other ways to keep the relationship interesting.

DOUBT: *He or she might think I am HIV-infected or have another STD if I suggest using a condom.*
DOUBT-BUSTER ACTION: I can say that I don't have anything infectious, but this is good protection anyway.

DOUBT: *It won't work if I don't do it right.*

DOUBT: *It might start an argument if I say no.*

DOUBT: *The condom might break.*

For the first four ideas, work with the class to generate the "doubt busters" that counter the "doubts" and then identify what can be said or done to improve the likelihood of success. Leave the rest of the ideas on the board.

2. Now repeat the exercise for abstinence. Ask students for doubts about their ability to stay abstinent in the face of the temptation to have sex. Many of the items may be similar to the ones you have already listed and will address issues such as: (1) I will seem inexperienced or silly; (2) he or she will think that I don't love him or her enough to do anything; (3) it might start an argument and hurt our relationship. Add these ideas to the list of doubts that you generated before.

3. Hand out **Sticking with Abstinence and Protection** (Worksheet 15.1) to each student. Explain that they are to choose two doubts about sticking with abstinence or protection and write them in the spaces on their worksheets. Have students work in pairs to help each other figure out ACTIONS to counter those doubts and strengthen their preparation for staying abstinent or using protection, and write these actions on their worksheets.

# Sticking with Abstinence and Protection

*Directions*: Write some DOUBTS that might make it harder for you to abstain or use protection. Then, pair up with a partner and write ACTIONS (DOUBT BUSTERS) that counter that DOUBT and make you even more prepared to get what you want.

DOUBT: ______________________________

______________________________

______________________________

______________________________

DOUBT-BUSTER ACTION: ______________________________

______________________________

______________________________

______________________________

DOUBT: ______________________________

______________________________

______________________________

______________________________

DOUBT-BUSTER ACTION: ______________________________

______________________________

______________________________

______________________________

# CLASS 16

## SKILLS INTEGRATION—IV

### SYNOPSIS

Through a discussion about sticking with choices and practice with a final role-playing situation, Class 16 provides an opportunity for students to extend skills learned for abstinence or avoiding unprotected intercourse.

### PREPARATION

- Review Appendix C, "How to Use Role Plays."
- Copy a classroom set of **A Love Story** (Handout 16.1) and **Being Careful on the Couch** (Role Play 16.3).
- Copy for each student **Chris and Pat** (Worksheet 16.2).
- Write on the board the incomplete "I Learned" statements.
- Copy for each student **Observer Checklist** (Form 16.4).
- *Optional:* Have ready *Refusals* and *Delaying Tactics* Posters and *Role Play Cards* from *Reducing the Risk Supplementary Kit.*

# OUTLINE OF ACTIVITIES

| Activity | Time | Materials |
| --- | --- | --- |
| Review HIV Homework | 5–10 minutes | **How HIV Would Change My Life** (Homework 12.2) previously completed |
| Chris and Pat | 15–25 minutes | **A Love Story** (Handout 16.1) **Chris and Pat** (Worksheet 16.2) |
| Role-Play in Small Groups | 20–25 minutes | **Being Careful on the Couch** (Role play 16.3) **Observer Checklist** (Form 16.4) *Refusals* and *Delaying Tactics* Posters, *Role Play Cards (optional)* |
| "I Learned" Statements | 5–15 minutes | Incomplete statements on the board. |

# ACTIVITIES

## Review STD Homework

Using their completed homework **How HIV Would Change My Life** (from Class 12), ask students to volunteer any ways that an STD infection would (1) require them to act differently, (2) harm them, or (3) make their lives more difficult.

## Chris and Pat

1. Introduce this activity by explaining to students that they will read a story about two young people who care about each other, then answer questions on a worksheet. Pass out **A Love Story** (Handout 16.1) and **Chris and Pat** (Worksheet 16.2). Tell students to think about the following as they listen to the story:
   a. Chris and Pat's reasons *for* having sex;
   b. their reasons for *not* having sex;
   c. what Chris and Pat *can do to make sure they don't have sex.*

2. Read the story aloud or have a student read it while the rest of the class follows along. Then have students answer questions 1 through 4 on **Chris and Pat** (Worksheet 16.2). After students have had a chance to answer the questions, review several answers to questions and write several students' responses on the board. Discuss responses as needed.

3. Explain to students that the last two questions on the worksheet are not about Chris and Pat, but about themselves. Have students complete these two questions based on what they think they would say or do. If time allows, ask students to share responses that may not have been discussed in class. Collect the copies of **A Love Story** (Handout 16.1) for use with other classes.

## Role-Play in Small Groups

1. Briefly describe the role play.

   *Optional:* Review the skills students have learned, using the *Refusals* and *Delaying Tactics* Posters from the Supplementary Kit.

2. Divide class into groups of no more than six with equal numbers of pairs. Provide copies of **Being Careful on the Couch** (Role Play 16.3) for each group.

3. As usual, instruct students to alternate roles in the unscripted part and to use **Observer Checklist** (Form 16.4). Move from group to group to help facilitate the discussion as needed.

   *Optional:* Pass out a set of *Role Play Cards* to each group. Ask each member to take one card. Review each role with the whole group. Write key words on the board:

   - Student Role Player #1: Read lines.
   - Student Role Player #2: Respond to lines.
   - Student Observer #1: Set the stage for the role play, and use **Observer Checklist** (Form 16.4)
   - Student Observer #2: Use **Observer Checklist** (Form 16.4) and lead small group discussion using the guidelines on the back of card.

## "I Learned" Statements

1. Explain that the purpose of the "I Learned" exercise is to help students focus on what has been most helpful or significant for them during this unit. Since they sometimes get a great deal of information at once, more than they can possibly remember, it can be advantageous to single out that which is most important.

2. Put the following incomplete sentences on the board. Ask the students to think about what they have just learned or relearned about sexuality, or about themselves or their values. Read the sentence stems and ask students to pick three and finish them on their own paper.

   | | |
   |---|---|
   | I learned that... | I was surprised that I... |
   | I noticed that I... | I was displeased that I... |
   | I discovered that I... | I was pleased that I... |

   *Optional:* Have students write out the "I Learned" statements and turn them in. The teacher should then just check to see that they were thoughtfully completed, and return them to students.

## Lesson and Course Summary

**Chris and Pat** (Worksheet 16.2) and "I Learned" provide an opportunity for students to review skills presented in the course and to think about what they have learned and what they may have discovered about themselves and their thoughts and actions on abstinence, sex and protection.

# A Love Story

Chris and Pat are sophomores. They've been going out for eight months and have a very special relationship. They spend a lot of time together and trust each other. They tell each other everything. In many ways, they are best friends.

At the beginning, they decided they didn't want to have sex. They haven't talked about it a lot but Chris believes it's worth it to save sex for marriage. Chris loves Pat a lot, but worries that their relationship would change if they have sex. Pat knows and respects Chris's feelings.

They haven't actually made love, though they do kiss and touch each other a lot and have gotten close to going all the way. Lately, Pat has been hearing that many of their friends are having sex. Pat feels a little jealous. Pat worries about "falling behind" other kids the same age and doesn't want to be a virgin forever.

So Pat has been putting some pressure on Chris to have sex, and they've started talking about it more. Pat is confused. On the one hand, Pat respects Chris's feelings and doesn't want to talk Chris into doing something Chris doesn't want to do. On the other hand, Pat doesn't think it's that important to wait for marriage. Their relationship has become a little tense. They argue more and Pat's talking more to other people and spending less time with Chris.

Chris worries about losing Pat and talked to a friend about these concerns. The friend said, "So what's the big deal? Having sex isn't that big a thing. You know everybody is doing it." Chris knows that isn't true but sometimes *feels* like the only one who isn't. "Maybe it isn't all that special," Chris thinks. "But, then again, maybe it is." Chris would like to talk to a parent about it, but doesn't know how Mom or Dad would react. So Chris feels pretty lost and doesn't know what to do.

Chris and Pat still spend some time together, and one Saturday night they go to the movies. After the movie, they decide to go back to Chris's house to talk. When they get there at around ten o'clock, they find out that Chris's parents have gone to a party and won't be back till much later. So Chris and Pat are alone in the house.

# Chris and Pat

*Directions:* After hearing the story of Chris and Pat, answer the first four questions. Don't answer questions 5 and 6 until the teacher tells you to.

1. Describe one important reason that Chris might not want to have sex.

   a. ______________________________

2. Describe two things that Chris can say or do to delay having sex.

   a. ______________________________

   b. ______________________________

3. Describe one reason why Pat would be better off waiting until Chris is ready.

   a. ______________________________

4. Describe two things Pat can do to help wait until Chris is ready.

   a. ______________________________

   b. ______________________________

5. Describe one reason that *you* might not want to have sex. I might not want to have sex because…

   a. ______________________________

6. Describe two things that *you* can say or do to delay having sex until you are ready.

   a. ______________________________

   b. ______________________________

# Being Careful on the Couch

*Setting the stage:*

You have decided that you don't want to have unprotected sex with your boyfriend or girlfriend. On this evening, you both have been watching TV. You decide to lie down on the couch together. You remember that this is exactly what happened the last two times you had sex without protection.

**Person 1:** I love you.

**Person 2:**

**Person 1:** Don't worry, baby.

**Person 2:**

**Person 1:** But I'm sure it's safe.

**Person 2:**

**Person 1:** Anyhow, nothing bad is going to happen to us. Believe me.

**Person 2:**

**Person 1:** Well, I just don't want to give this up—it's too much fun.

**Person 2:**

**Person 1:** I promise we'll go get some protection for next time.

**Person 2:**

**Person 1:** What's wrong? Why change a good thing?

**Person 2:**

Name: ______________________________ Date: ______________________________

# Observer Checklist

ROLE PLAY #

| REFUSALS | 1 | 2 | 3 | 4 | 5 | 6 |
|---|---|---|---|---|---|---|
| Said "NO" | | | | | | |
| Body Language Said "NO" | | | | | | |
| Repeated Refusal | | | | | | |
| Suggested Alternative | | | | | | |
| Built the Relationship | | | | | | |
| DELAYING TACTICS | | | | | | |
| Used Delay Statement | | | | | | |
| Used Delay Action | | | | | | |
| Created Space | | | | | | |
| Ended the Situation Quickly | | | | | | |
| Built the Relationship | | | | | | |

# REFERENCES


Abbey, N., and E. Wagman. 1987. *Saying no to alcohol.* Santa Cruz, CA: ETR Associates.

Alan Guttmacher Institute. 1994. *Sex and America's Teenagers.* New York.

Barth, R. P. 1986. *Social and cognitive treatment of children and adolescents.* San Francisco: Jossey-Bass.

Barth, R. P., and Derezotes, D. S. 1990. *Preventing adolescent abuse: Effective intervention strategies and techniques.* Lexington, MA: Lexington.

Barth, R. P., K. Middleton and E. Wagman. 1989. A social and cognitive skill-building approach to preventing teenage pregnancy. *Theory into Practice:*28.

Barth, R. P., S. P. Schinke and J. Maxwell. 1985. Coping skills training for school-age mothers. *Journal of Social Service Research* 8:75-94.

Bignell, S. 1982. *Sex education: Teacher's guide and resource manual.* Santa Cruz, CA: ETR Associates.

Centers for Disease Control and Prevention. 1994. Pregnancy, sexually transmitted diseases, and related risk behaviors among U.S. adolescents. Adolescent Health: State of the Nation monograph series, no. 2. CDC Publication No. 099-4630. Atlanta, GA.

Centers for Disease Control and Prevention. 1993. Update: Barrier protection against HIV infection and other sexually transmitted diseases. *Morbidity and Mortality Weekly Report* 42:589-591.

Centers for Disease Control and Prevention. 1988. Condoms for prevention of sexually transmitted diseases. *Morbidity and Mortality Weekly Report* 37:132-137.

Elam, S. M., L. C. Rose and A. M. Gallup. 1992. The 24th annual Gallup/Phi Delta Kappa poll of the public's attitudes toward the public schools. *Phi Delta Kappan* 73 (1): 41-53.

Gilchrist, L. D., and S. P. Schinke. 1983. Coping with contraception: Cognitive and behavioral methods with adolescents. *Cognitive Therapy and Research* 7:379-388.

Harris, L. 1988. *Public attitudes toward teenage pregnancy, sex education and birth control.* New York: Planned Parenthood Federation of America.

Hatcher, R., J. Trussel, F. Stewart et al. 1994. *Contraceptive Technology.* 16th ed. New York: Irvington Publishers, Inc.

Hofferth, S. L., J. R. Kahn and W. Baldwin. 1987. Premarital sexual activity among U.S. teenage women over the past three decades. *Family Planning Perspectives* 19:46-53.

Quackenbush, M., and P. Sargent. 1988. *Teaching AIDS: A resource guide on Acquired Immune Deficiency Syndrome.* Santa Cruz, CA: ETR Associates.

Scales, P. C., and M. R. Roper. 1994. Challenges to sexuality education in the schools. In *The sexuality education challenge: Promoting healthy sexuality in young people,* ed. J. C. Drolet and K. Clark, 69-90. Santa Cruz, CA: ETR Associates.

Stout, J. W., and F. P. Rivara. 1989. Schools and sex education: Does it work? *Pediatrics* 83:375-379.

Trussell, J. 1988. Teenage pregnancy in the United States. *Family Planning Perspectives* 20:262-272.

# APPENDIX A

# *Reducing the Risk Supplementary Kit* Correlation

| Kit Materials | Related Lessons |
|---|---|
| **Posters** | |
| • Refusals | 3, 4, 10, 14, 16 |
| • Delaying Tactics | 5, 10, 14, 16 |
| • Ground Rules | Prior to 1 |
| • Signs of Sex, Signs of Caution<br>Yellow Alert Signs<br>Red Alert Signs | 6 |
| **Traffic Light Cards**<br>• Red Light Signal<br>• Green Light Signal<br>• Yellow Light Signal | 13 |
| **Risk Behavior Cards** | 13 |
| **Role Play Cards** | 1, 3, 4, 5, 9, 10, 11, 14, 16 |

# APPENDIX B

# Questions and Answers on *Reducing the Risk*

## Research Questions

**1. Are there plans for more research on *Reducing the Risk* (*RTR*)?**

ETR Associates currently has no plans to further evaluate *RTR*. However, we are developing and evaluating new curricula based upon *RTR*. In one current project, we have expanded *RTR* to twenty sessions, divided it equally into sequential ninth grade and tenth grade curricula, added a peer component, and made other changes. These ninth and tenth grade curricula are being rigorously evaluated as part of a larger more comprehensive HIV, STD and pregnancy prevention project in twenty schools in California and Texas. In another project, we are developing a curriculum primarily for Hispanic youth that is based upon the principles of *RTR*. It will be rigorously evaluated.

**2. Did *RTR* affect the use of contraception/protection among those students already sexually active?**

About two-thirds of the students in the study had not initiated intercourse prior to *RTR*. *RTR* had its clearest and most dramatic impact upon this group; it substantially reduced unprotected intercourse, mostly by delaying the onset of intercourse and partly by increasing the use of protection.

About one-third (37%) of the students had initiated intercourse prior to the program. In part because of the smaller sample size, it was more difficult to determine the impact of *RTR* upon contraceptive use in this sample. For the entire sample of youth who had initiated intercourse prior to the program, there were no statistically significant differences in the increase in contraceptive use between the *RTR* group and the control group. On some measures of contraceptive use, the *RTR* group did report greater increases in contraceptive use than did the control group, but these increases were not statistically significant.

However, among females and lower-risk youth who had initiated intercourse prior to the program, the *RTR* group had statistically significant greater increases in contraceptive use than did the control group.

Thus, these data provided some evidence that *RTR* had a positive impact upon contraceptive use among sexually experienced students. However, because of the inconsistency among the findings and because of the relatively small sample sizes, this evidence is less compelling than the data for the impact of *RTR* on youth not sexually experienced before *RTR*.

**3. Would the research results change with the newer editions of *RTR*?**

The first edition focused primarily, but not entirely, upon pregnancy prevention and had a greater effect upon females. The second and third editions give more emphasis to STD, HIV and condoms and, thus, may have a greater impact upon males.

Because nothing was removed from the curriculum, all of the positive effects observed in the first edition should also be produced by the second and third editions.

**4. In the research, did students include anal intercourse in their concept of "sexual intercourse"?**

Because the first edition focused more upon pregnancy prevention, questionnaires used in the research defined sexual intercourse as "placing a male's penis in a female's vagina."

# Implementation Questions

**1. If *RTR* is more effective with kids not yet sexually active, wouldn't *RTR* be better for middle school students?**

*RTR* did significantly delay the onset of intercourse and appears to be more effective with students who had not yet initiated intercourse. Thus, ideally it should be implemented before more than 20% to 40% of the students have initiated intercourse.

In some communities, this means it should be implemented in middle school; in other communities with a lower rate of middle school sexual activity, it should be implemented in the ninth or tenth grades.

For at least two reasons, the curriculum is also an appropriate curriculum for sexually active youth. First, *RTR* helps students say no to unwanted intercourse, and all youth, even sexually active youth, sometimes need the skills to avoid intercourse. Second, the curriculum did have positive effects upon contraceptive use among some groups of sexually active youth.

**2. Do I have to teach all the lessons? If I don't have time for them all, what can be dropped?**

To the best of our knowledge, the effectiveness of the curriculum is not dependent upon any single activity. Thus, if any single activity is dropped, most of the effectiveness will probably be maintained. On the other hand, if the curriculum is shortened by 25% or 50%, then the effectiveness probably will be diminished. From our research, we simply cannot determine which activities are the most critical.

If teachers must drop some of the activities, then they might use the following principle: if most of the students have not had sexual intercourse, then some of the activities on protection and contraception might be condensed or dropped.

**3. How much flexibility do I have to change any lesson?**

For the evaluation, teachers implemented the curriculum with a high degree of fidelity. Thus, to increase the chances of effectiveness, the curriculum should not be significantly changed.

However, given that caveat, it is probably true that the effectiveness of the curriculum will not be diminished if minor changes are made, and perhaps some minor changes might increase its effectiveness for a particular group of students. For example, if the scripts in the role plays sound stilted to a particular group of students, rewriting them so that they still illustrate the same communication skills but use words more appropriate for a particular audience may improve the effectiveness for that audience. Similarly, if students have lots of questions about an important topic, then spending a little more time on that topic and a little less time on another may be appropriate.

On the other hand, we do not recommend dropping activities, especially the role plays, or significantly changing the activities.

### 4. How can I make *RTR* more culturally inclusive?

During the development and piloting of the *RTR* curriculum, reactions of teenagers from diverse backgrounds were critical to the completion of the final product. Several steps were taken to ensure that the curriculum addressed their needs. First, four multi-racial focus groups of tenth graders in urban, suburban and rural communities were questioned about ways to make the exercises more fitting and effective. These groups also generated ideas for new activities. Information gleaned from these teen consultants was incorporated into all aspects of the curriculum: the vignettes, role plays, classroom activities and homework assignments.

After input from the four focus groups, the curriculum was pilot tested in five diverse schools. The schools included two continuation school classes, an English as a Second Language class, and classes in suburban, rural and inner-city schools. Extensive revisions were completed following the pilot.

All of the above steps were implemented in order to make *RTR* as culturally sensitive and inclusive as possible. However, the developers understand that no curriculum can be perfectly relevant to every group or community. Therefore, the most effective way to make *RTR* culturally relevant for specific groups of students is to involve them in the revision of the scripted role play scenarios. These revisions can be done by a culturally representative group of peer educators or by an individual class.

*Important Note:* Fidelity to the curriculum can be maintained only if the revised scenarios teach the skills identified in the lesson (e.g. refusals, delaying tactics) and if the type of role play used in the lesson is kept the same (e.g. scripted, partially scripted, nonscripted).

### 5. How was *RTR* taught in the research study?

*RTR* was implemented in 15 consecutive days over a three-week period. It is probably acceptable to implement *RTR* two or three times per week and spread it over six weeks. We do not recommend implementing it only one time per week, because it may lose its continuity and students may forget too much between classes.

### 6. Can I teach the curriculum without using role plays?

No, unless you are willing to sacrifice its effectiveness. We believe that the role plays are among the most important activities in the curriculum. They reinforce important norms; they teach skills; they increase students' self-efficacy in using these skills; and they keep students experientially involved in the curriculum.

### 7. How can I tie *RTR* into Comprehensive School Health Education?

*RTR* is a prevention curriculum designed to reduce the behaviors that put young people at risk for pregnancy, STD and HIV. Prevention education differs from general health or sexuality education in that it has a clear prevention message that supports, models and reinforces a desired behavior. For example, the message in *RTR* is to avoid unprotected sex. The behaviors modeled, practiced and reinforced are (1) ways to successfully postpone sexual involvement, and (2) the use of protection for those who decide to be sexually active. Both the message and the behavioral practice help set a social norm of protection from pregnancy, STD and HIV.

In order to maintain *RTR*'s effectiveness as a prevention curriculum, it needs to be taught as a unit. As a unit, *RTR* can easily be inserted into a health framework where HIV and pregnancy prevention would be taught to adolescents. If refusals or delaying tactics have been taught previously in the health framework, those skills can be reviewed when teaching *RTR*. However, teachers need to be sure to include all the practice lessons in *RTR* because research tells us that students don't easily transfer skills from one type of situation to another. For example, they may learn to say no to tobacco but not use these same refusal skills when faced with a sexual situation.

**8. In Class 1, does the "statistical inaccuracy" of the number of pregnancies in a year invalidate the lesson? Returning slips of paper to the hat would yield more statistically accurate results.**

The purpose of the activity is not to demonstrate statistical risk, but to personalize the substantial risk of pregnancy with unprotected sexual intercourse. The "statistical inaccuracy" does not diminish the activity's effectiveness. The activity would be more statistically accurate if the slips of paper were returned to the hat after each drawing. This would allow some students to get pregnant two or more times in the same year, and would acknowledge that some students will not get pregnant in a year, even if they have unprotected intercourse each month. However, there is a concern that students who do not "get pregnant" during the activity may fail to personalize the risk of unprotected intercourse, which is the main purpose of the activity.

**9. How can we get administrative and community support to teach the "Protection Homework" assignments in Classes 7 and 8?**

The most effective method for gaining administrative support for the "Protection Homework" assignments is to inform administrators early about the goals and objectives of the entire curriculum, including the purpose of the Protection Shopping and Call/Visit a Clinic assignments. While many of the lessons in *RTR* focus on abstinence, some lessons focus on protection, and Classes 7 and 8 are particularly important because the purpose of both assignments is to provide students with practice in obtaining protection before they find themselves in a risky situation. This practice feels safe for the student because it is an "assignment." In addition, the practice can increase students' comfort with the steps to getting protection. Then, when they become sexually active, there will be an increased likelihood that they will use protection and avoid risks that may result in pregnancy or HIV or other STD infection.

While the lack of administrative and community support may be related to an assumption that assignments like these encourage students to become more sexually active, the research shows that this is not the case. In fact, this curriculum delayed the onset of sexual intercourse among students in the research study. In addition, it is helpful to assure administrators that this curriculum can be optional for students whose parents do not want them to participate in it.

It has been ETR Associates' experience that parental involvement early in the planning process is the easiest way to get parent and community support for any health or sexuality curriculum. We recommend that schools establish a health and sexuality education parent advisory committee and provide parent preview sessions.

The parent advisory committee can provide support by reviewing and approving the curriculum and can respond to parent and community concerns if they arise.

The parent preview sessions provide an opportunity for parents to meet the teacher and better understand the rationale and teaching approach used in all lessons.

Details about how to form and use advisory committees and how to be successful at hosting parent preview sessions can be found in *Step by Step to Comprehensive School Health: The Program Planning Guide* by William M. Kane, PhD, CHES, published by ETR Associates.

### 10. How do we deal with the issue of homosexuality in the context of teaching *RTR*?

*RTR* does not address homosexuality directly because the purpose of HIV prevention education is to reduce risky behavior, not to teach about a sexual orientation or lifestyle. Sometimes students make the assumption that only gay people can get HIV. It is important for a teacher to emphasize that this assumption is not based on facts.

Unprotected sexual intercourse and other risky sexual behaviors put people at risk for HIV infection. Anyone can become infected. In order to eliminate or reduce risk, everyone needs to avoid risk taking behaviors, which include unprotected sexual intercourse. In addition to emphasizing that behaviors put people at risk, the teacher should use gender neutral language when discussing relationships. For example, instead of saying "boyfriend" or "girlfriend," terms including "partner," "people we date," and "someone we are attracted to" can be more inclusive. When talking about intercourse, say "when a couple has sex." When talking about protection say "when a person removes his penis from the other partner" instead of "when a man removes his penis from the woman." It is important to use language and examples that all students can relate to, and to avoid reinforcing assumptions that all students are heterosexual.

### 11. How do we deal with the issue of sexual abuse, assault and rape in the context of *RTR*?

Issues of sexual abuse, assault and rape (including date rape) should be covered as part of a broader health and sexuality education program. Students should be taught that these forms of behavior are illegal, and teachers should make sure that students understand their rights, as well as reporting mechanisms and local resources available to victims of sexual abuse, assault and rape.

In the context of *RTR*, the teaching of refusals can be related to these issues. It is important to emphasize that students learn how to say "no" effectively and that refusals are to be honored. Teachers should reinforce the message that no one has the right to force or coerce others into sexual behavior against their will.

### 12. Do teachers really have to be trained to teach *RTR*?

Research has taught us that teachers are much more effective at implementing a new curriculum if they have received training in the content and the specific skills necessary to teach the program (Showers, 1993). In addition, *RTR* requires that teachers have well-developed facilitation skills to be able to deal effectively and comfortably with the sensitive subject matter addressed in the curriculum. Teachers usually need special training to develop these skills with comfort. Finally, teachers often need assistance in effectively implementing the many role plays in the curriculum (Weil, 1985). Training can provide them with a model for, and an opportunity to practice, teaching the role play lessons. As one teacher commented, "I usually have trouble with role plays but the steps are broken down to such a degree that I think these will really work." Another responded by saying, "I liked seeing the lessons modeled and having a chance to practice."

**13. What kinds of technical assistance and support can ETR Associates offer as teachers implement *RTR*?**

ETR Associates can provide several types of technical assistance to teachers as they implement *RTR*. Contact the Training Department at (408) 438-4060 for specific information.

# APPENDIX C

# How to Use Role Plays

The *Reducing the Risk* curriculum focuses on skill development, providing students practice in important skills they will need to make healthful decisions related to sex. The following provides specific and indepth process steps for practicing the refusals and delaying tactics used in the curriculum.

## Model the Skill with Scripted Role Plays

1. Select students who are comfortable reading in front of the class and who are mature enough to handle dialog about sexuality without experiencing a lot of embarrassment.
2. Ask remaining students to act as observers of the role play. Assign each of the behaviors to 5 or 6 students. Ask these students to notice if their assigned behavior is used during the role play.
3. Read the situation aloud and have selected students read the scripted role play.
4. Conduct large group discussion.
   a) Ask role players to comment on how they felt playing their roles and how they might feel if this was a real-life situation.
   b) Ask how these feelings might affect their use of refusals or delaying tactics.
   c) Ask the observers for their reactions to the role play and to identify how the skill was practiced.

## Role Play Skill Practice

1. *Phase One:* Prepare Small Groups for Role Play Practice
   a) Divide students into groups of four (equal numbers of males and females when possible).
   b) Identify roles (Person 1, Person 2, Observer, etc.) and instruct students to decide who will play which role in the first round, second round, etc.
   c) Prepare students for the observer roles by asking one Observer to set the stage for the role play and the other to lead the small group discussion. Both Observers should use the **Observer Checklist** to indicate behaviors demonstrated.
   d) Use a management tool such as instruction cards to assign roles and help keep students on task in their small groups. (A set of *Role Play Cards* is provided in the *Reducing the Risk Supplemental Kit.*)

2. *Phase Two:* Small Groups Act Out Role Plays

    a) Walk around the room and gather data about how students are using the skill. Use this data in the discussion phase.

    b) While walking from group to group, offer coaching if students are stuck or clearly practicing the skill incorrectly.

    c) Time each round of practice and tell students when to pass their cards for the next round. Once students become familiar with the process, you can drop this step.

3. *Phase Three:* Small Group Discussion

    Instruct students to discuss the following after each role play:

    a) Debrief feelings on how each person experienced his or her role (Person 1, Person 2, Observers).

    b) Using the checklist, Observers give feedback on how the skill was demonstrated. Encourage them to identify the behaviors that illustrated the skill was being practiced.

    c) Discuss any behaviors that weren't practiced and why they may have been omitted.

    d) Record any questions for large group discussion.

4. *Phase Four:* Large Group Discussion

    a) Identify feelings that came up about using the skill during the practice, including what was easy and what was difficult about practicing the skill.

    b) Ask if the Observers saw any behaviors that took away from the effectiveness of the skill (e.g., giggling, saying I'm sorry, etc.).

    c) Discuss how this situation was or wasn't similar to real life.

    d) Discuss any barriers to using the skill, helping students identify ways to overcome these barriers.

    e) If students feel the situation isn't like real life, have them rewrite the situation and scripted dialog so that it is.

    f) Discuss any questions students identified in their small group discussion.

5. *Phase Five:* Personalize Experiences and Generalize

    a) Ask what left the biggest impression with students as a result of the role play.

    b) Ask students to identify how they will use the skill in the next week or two with their friends.

# APPENDIX D

# Skills Overview

## Refusals

*Purpose:* A way of communicating that lets us effectively say no to things we do not want to do, such as taking sexual risks.

| Behavior | Actions* | Examples |
|---|---|---|
| **1. Say "No!"** | Use the word "no." | "No, I don't want to do that." |
| | Don't laugh, look away, make excuses or explain. | Look straight at the other person with a serious look on your face. |
| **2. Repeat the refusal.** | Use broken record by repeating original "no" statement until other person stops pressuring. | "No, I don't want to do that. No, I don't want to do that. No, I don't want to do that." |
| | Restate "no," increasing intensity by including: | |
| | • statements about how the situation makes you feel | "No, and when you pressure me I feel angry." |
| | • adding consequences if the situation doesn't change | "No, and if you keep pressuring me I'm going to leave." |
| **3. Suggest an alternative.** | Suggest another activity that is realistic and appealing. | "Let's go to a movie, for a walk, to a friend's, etc." |
| | Suggest another activity that gets you out of the situation. | "Let's go to a movie, for a walk, to a friend's, etc." |
| | Move toward acting on the alternative. | Get the paper to see what is at the movies, start on a walk together, call friends to see if they're home. |

*(continued...)*

# Refusals *(continued)*

| Behavior | Actions* | Examples |
|---|---|---|
| **4. Use body language that says "No!"** | firm voice | Use a strong, business-like tone. |
| | serious expression | "I mean it" look on face. |
| | eye contact | Look directly at the person's face. |
| | soldier body | Stand up straight and confident. |
| | gestures that emphasize point | Use hand, arm movement to emphasize point. |
| | Body says the same thing as your words. | Look serious when you say no. |
| | Fight back as last resort. | Push someone away. |
| **5. Build the relationship (if appropriate).** | Strong, honest communication. | "I want you to stop that." |
| | Use I-statements. | "I feel mad when you push me to do things I'm not ready for." |
| | Accept and acknowledge other's needs and wants. | "I want to be with you too." |
| | Talk and act in a way that says you want to keep the relationship going. | "I don't want to have sex with you but I do want to keep seeing you and being close." |

* It is not necessary for all actions to be present to implement the skill effectively.

# Delaying Tactics

*Purpose:* A way of communicating that is an effective alternative to directly saying no and that can buy time until we can think about how to communicate what we really want.

| Behavior | Actions | Examples |
|---|---|---|
| **1. Make a delay statement.** | Stall for time. | "I'll have to think about this." |
| | Make an excuse. | "I'm really not feeling well." |
| | Question what is going on. | "What are you doing?" |
| | Change the subject. | "Did you see 'Martin' last night?" |
| | Excuse yourself from the situation. | "Sorry, I have to go." |
| | Pretend request isn't serious. | "You're kidding, right?" |
| **2. Take a delay action.** | Change what you are doing. | Stop kissing. Get up and get something to eat. |
| | Act distracted. | Look around. Pretend you've lost something. |
| | Drop something. | Drop your keys. |
| | Become physically unable to respond. | Start coughing and ask for water. Get a sudden pain. |
| | Leave the situation. | Go to the restroom. Go get some fresh air. |
| **3. Create space.** | Use body language. | Serious expression. Look directly at the person. Arms in front of body. Gestures that emphasize your point. |
| | Move away. | Take a step back. Turn away. |
| **4. End the situation quickly.** | Leave the scene. | "Got to go, I'm late!" "I just remembered something." |
| | Fight back as last resort. | Push the person away. |
| **5. Build the relationship (if appropriate).** | Strong, honest communication. | "I want you to stop that." |
| | Use I-statements. | "I feel nervous when you push me to do things I'm not ready for." |
| | Accept and acknowledge other's needs and wants. | "I want to be with you too." |
| | Talk and act in a way that says you want to keep the relationship going. | "I don't want to have sex with you but I do want to keep seeing you and being close." |

# APPENDIX E

# Answering Student Questions

## Using a Question Box

Anonymous Question Boxes are used in prevention education classes to provide an opportunity for students to ask questions about sensitive issues that they might be too embarrassed to ask aloud. Here are some guidelines for using this technique.

1. Validate students' concerns about asking questions.
   - Introduce the box by telling students that people of all ages have questions about sexual activity and STD, including HIV. Sometimes these questions are never answered because people aren't given the opportunity to ask, or because they're too embarrassed to ask. Here's your opportunity to do so anonymously.
   - Remind students that there is no such thing as a dumb question.
   - To prevent those students with pressing questions from feeling uncomfortable, ask all students to write something on a slip of paper. It may be a question they don't feel comfortable asking in class, feedback on how the unit is going, or input about some topic they want covered.
2. Reinforce or add appropriate ground rules.
   - **Confidentiality:** This is a confidential activity. Students should not put their names on the papers.
   - **Right to Pass:** All questions are OK, except questions about the teacher's or other students' personal life. Let students know that you may choose not to answer a question in class, not because the question is a bad question, but because you're not ready to answer it for any one of these reasons:
     - You may think it is not of interest to all students.
     - You're not prepared to lead a class discussion around it.
     - The topic may be covered later in the unit.
     - You feel too uncomfortable answering it.

     Suggest students see you at the end of class if their question isn't answered so that you can try to answer it privately.
   - **Language:** Tell students that you are trying to balance two goals: to teach the medical vocabulary for body parts and functions, and to communicate with them so that they understand. If students do not know the medical word for something they have a question about, they should use whatever word they know. You will answer using the medical word.
3. Give yourself permission to not be perfect.
   - Collect questions at the end of class so you have time to review and practice answering them.

- If you don't know the answer, it's OK to say, "I don't know," and refer students to another source, or do more research when you have time.
- Don't be afraid to revise your answer. You will sometimes make mistakes or have second thoughts about your answers. Be honest and provide the right answer as soon as possible.
- If you feel uncomfortable with a question, tell the class. Students will respect that and may be relieved to find out that other people sometimes feel embarrassed to talk about sex.

## Finding the Meaning Behind Questions

As you review and prepare to answer student questions about sensitive topics such as sexual behavior, use the following guidelines to form answers that are accurate, appropriate and complete. Questions may be grouped into five broad categories, which of course overlap:

1. Requests for information.
2. "Am I Normal?" questions.
3. "Permission-seeking" questions.
4. Questions used to shock the teacher and the rest of the class.
5. Questions about teacher's personal beliefs.

### Requests for Information

If you know the answer, fine. If not, it's OK to say, "I don't know," and then refer the student to an appropriate source. If there are some values issues within the context of the question, make sure various points of view are presented.

Sometimes a question, although informational, is one that you consider inappropriate for classroom discussion. Problems can be avoided if you establish in the class ground rules an agreement such as: "All questions are valid. However, I will have to make the final decision about the appropriateness of each question for class discussion. If you turn in a question anonymously which I choose not to answer, it is not because it is a bad question. I may feel that it is not of interest to all students or that I am not prepared to lead a class discussion around that issue. Please see me at the end of class if ever this happens so that I can try to answer your question privately."

### "Am I Normal?" Questions

These questions generally focus on adolescents' concerns about their bodies and the emotional and physical changes of puberty. Be sure to:

- Validate student concerns (e.g., "Many young people worry that...") and provide information about what they can expect to happen during the adolescent years.
- Refer students to parents, clergy, family physician, community resources or school counselor for further discussion, if appropriate.

## Permission-Seeking Questions

These come in two common forms, and may be asking your permission to, or not to, participate in a particular behavior (e.g., "Is it normal to...?" or "Did you...when you were growing up?").

Avoid the use of the word "normal" when answering these questions. Normal for some is morally unsanctionable for others. Present what is known medically, legally, etc. (the facts), and discuss the moral, religious and emotional implications, making sure all points of view are covered. Refer students to parents and clergy for discussion of moral/religious questions.

It is also important to establish, in the context of class ground rules, an agreement related to discussion of personal behavior, such as: "No discussion of personal behavior during class." If and when you get a question about your personal behavior, you can remind students of this ground rule and redirect the discussion to the pros and cons (religious, moral, medical, emotional, legal, interpersonal, etc.) of the particular behavior in question. Again, refer students to parents and clergy for further discussion of moral/religious questions.

## Shock Questions

If you deem the question inappropriate for classroom discussion, again refer to the ground rule related to appropriate questions for classroom discussion. Offer to answer the question privately. Taking "shock" questions seriously is one way to defuse them.

Sometimes the shock comes not from the content of the question, but the vocabulary utilized. You can re-word the question to defuse it, especially if you have previously established a ground rule related to vocabulary, such as, "In this class, I want to teach the proper vocabulary for body parts and functions, and I also want to communicate with you. Sometimes you may not know the correct word for something you have a question about. Use whatever word you know to ask that question and I will answer using the correct (acceptable) word."

## Personal Beliefs

Teachers' opinions about how or whether to respond to these questions differ. Some feel it is important to respond, while others believe their role as teacher gives their response too much weight. If you share your opinion, emphasize that it is only one of many and recommend that students ask their parents about family values and beliefs. Avoid sharing information about personal sexual practices.

# APPENDIX F

# Condom Use Effectiveness

## Condoms and Their Use in Preventing HIV Infection and Other STDs*

With more than 1 million Americans infected with HIV, most of them through sexual transmission, and an estimated 12 million other sexually transmitted diseases occurring each year in the United States, effective strategies for preventing these diseases are critical.

The proper and consistent use of latex condoms when engaging in sexual intercourse—vaginal, anal or oral—can greatly reduce a person's risk of acquiring or transmitting STDs, including HIV infection. In fact, *recent studies provide compelling evidence that latex condoms are highly effective in protecting against HIV infection when used properly for every act of intercourse.*

The protection that proper use of latex condoms provides against HIV transmission is most evident from studies of couples in which one member is infected with HIV and the other is not, i.e., "discordant couples." In a study of discordant couples in Europe, among 123 couples who reported consistent condom use, none of the uninfected partners became infected. In contrast, among the 122 couples who used condoms *inconsistently,* 12 of the uninfected partners became infected.

As these studies indicate, condoms must be used *consistently* and *correctly* to provide maximum protection. *Consistent* use means using a condom from start to finish with each act of intercourse. *Correct condom use* should include the following steps:

- Use a new condom for each act of intercourse.
- Put on the condom as soon as erection occurs and before any sexual contact (vaginal, anal or oral).
- Hold the tip of the condom and unroll it onto the erect penis, leaving space at the tip of the condom, yet ensuring that no air is trapped in the condom's tip.
- Adequate lubrication is important, but use only water-based lubricants, such as glycerin or lubricating jellies (which can be purchased at any pharmacy). Oil-based lubricants, such as petroleum jelly, cold cream, hand lotion or baby oil, can weaken the condom.
- Withdraw from the partner immediately after ejaculation, holding the condom firmly to keep it from slipping off.

## Myths About Condoms

There continues to be misinformation and misunderstanding about condom effectiveness. The Centers for Disease Control and Prevention (CDC) provides the following updated

*Reprinted from *CDC HIV/AIDS Prevention Fact Sheet,* 30 July 1993. Atlanta, GA: Centers for Disease Control and Prevention information to address some common myths about condoms. This information is based on findings from recent epidemiologic, laboratory and clinical studies.

- **Myth #1: Condoms don't work.**

Some persons have expressed concern about studies that report failure rates among couples using condoms for pregnancy prevention. Analysis of these studies indicates that the large range of efficacy rates is related to incorrect or inconsistent use. The fact is latex condoms are highly effective for pregnancy prevention, but only when they are used properly. Research indicates that only 30 to 60 percent of men who claim to use condoms for contraception actually use them for every act of intercourse. Further, even people who use condoms every time may not use them correctly. Incorrect use contributes to the possibility that the condom could leak from the base or break.

- **Myth #2: HIV can pass through condoms.**

A commonly held misperception is that latex condoms contain "holes" that allow passage of HIV. Although this may be true for natural membrane condoms, laboratory studies show that intact latex condoms provide a continuous barrier to microorganisms, including HIV, as well as sperm.

- **Myth #3: Condoms frequently break.**

Another area of concern expressed by some is about the quality of latex condoms. Condoms are classified as medical devices and are regulated by the FDA. Every latex condom manufactured in the United States is tested for defects before it is packaged. During the manufacturing process, condoms are double-dipped in latex and undergo stringent quality control procedures. Several studies clearly show that condom breakage rates in this country are less than 2 percent. Most of the breakage is due to incorrect usage rather than poor condom quality. Using oil-based lubricants can weaken latex, causing the condom to break. In addition, condoms can be weakened by exposure to heat or sunlight or by age, or they can be torn by teeth or fingernails.

## Preventing HIV Infection and Other STDs

### Recommended Prevention Strategies

Abstaining from sexual activity is the most effective HIV prevention strategy. However, for individuals who choose to be sexually active, the following are highly effective:

- Engaging in sexual activities that do not involve vaginal, anal or oral intercourse.
- Having intercourse only with one uninfected partner.
- Using latex condoms correctly from start to finish with each act of intercourse.

### Other HIV Prevention Strategies

- ***Condoms for Women***

The FDA recently approved a female condom, which will soon be available in the United States. [The female condom is now available—Ed.] A limited study of this condom as a contraceptive indicates a failure rate of about 26 percent in 1 year. Although laboratory studies indicate that the device serves as a mechanical barrier to viruses, further clinical research is necessary to determine its effectiveness in preventing transmission of HIV.

- ***Spermicides***

The role of spermicides in preventing HIV infection is uncertain. Condoms lubricated with spermicides are not likely to be more effective than condoms used with other water-based lubricants. Spermicides added to the tip of the condom are also not likely to add protection against HIV.

### Making Responsible Choices

In summary, sexually transmitted diseases, including HIV infection, are preventable, and individuals have several responsible prevention strategies to choose from. But the effectiveness of each one depends largely on the individual. Those who practice abstinence as a prevention strategy will find it effective only if they always abstain. Similarly, those who choose any of the other recommended prevention strategies, including condoms, will find them highly effective if used correctly and consistently.

# Questions and Answers: *MMWR* on the Effectiveness of Condoms*

**1. What about studies that suggest condoms have as high as a 15.7% contraceptive failure rate?**

These studies do not distinguish between inconsistent and consistent condom use. Recent studies show that pregnancy rates are estimated to be as low as 2% for couples who use condoms consistently and correctly (Trussell et al., 1991). Similarly, in two studies involving extremely high-risk couples in which one partner was HIV-infected and the other was not, condoms were found to be highly effective when used consistently and correctly.

**2. What does "highly effective" mean?**

We know from the discordant couple studies that in extreme risk situations the consistent use of condoms provides a significant reduction in risk. (See p. 233.)

**3. Isn't it naive to think that people can use condoms consistently and correctly?**

No, people can use condoms correctly by following a few simple steps. Discordant couple studies clearly demonstrate that consistent and correct condom use is possible if the couple is highly motivated.

**4. Can't condoms break?**

Condoms rarely break. In those cases where breakage occurs, it is usually related to user error rather than condom quality. Using old condoms is a leading cause of breakage. Other common reasons for breakage include fingernail tears, exposure to heat or sunlight, reusing condoms, or unrolling the condom before putting it on.

---

*Reprinted from *Background Information on the Morbidity and Mortality Weekly Report: The Effectiveness of Condoms.* Information Kit. Atlanta, GA: U.S. Department of Health and Human Services, Public Health Service, Centers for Disease Control and Prevention.

Use of oil-based lubricants such as baby oil, vegetable oil, petroleum jelly and cold cream can weaken latex condoms considerably and cause them to break. Mineral oil, a common ingredient of hand lotions, can cause a 90% decrease in condom strength after as little as 60 seconds of exposure (Voeller et al., 1989).

**5. How are condoms regulated and tested?**

Condoms are classified as medical devices, regulated by the FDA, and manufactured according to national standards. Every condom sold in the United States is tested by the manufacturer electronically for defects, including holes or areas of thinning, before it is packaged. During the manufacturing process, condoms undergo stringent quality testing.

In addition, the FDA randomly tests condoms using the water-leak test, in which a condom is filled with 300 ml of water. If the FDA finds that more than four per 1000 condoms leak, the lot is not allowed to be sold here.

**6. Don't condoms have microscopic holes that allow HIV to pass through?**

Condoms are required to undergo demanding tests, including tests for holes before they are sold. If any holes are found, the condoms are discarded. Laboratory studies show that intact latex condoms provide a continuous barrier to microorganisms as well as sperm.

**7. Researchers studying surgical gloves made out of latex found "channels of 5 microns that penetrated the entire thickness of the glove."**

The quality of latex condoms is higher than that of latex gloves. Condoms are made differently than gloves. Condoms are double-dipped in latex while gloves are only single-dipped. Condoms also undergo much more stringent quality control procedures than gloves.

**8. What about a University of Texas Medical Branch study that estimated condoms to be only 69% effective in preventing HIV in heterosexual couples?**

The University of Texas did not conduct a new study, but rather a meta-analysis of existing studies. That is, it applied statistical methods to previously published studies. This method has several flaws. First, the study only cites data collected prior to July 1990, overlooking recent studies that provide some of the most compelling evidence that condoms are effective. Second, the study did not distinguish between consistent and inconsistent use of condoms.

**9. Why did the FDA approve the female condom if it has proven to be only 74% effective in recent studies?**

The female condom is the first barrier method of contraception available within the control of the female partner which provides some level of protection against pregnancy and STD, including HIV. As a very new product, limited studies have been conducted on its effectiveness against STD and HIV. However, the clinical data do suggest that female condoms provide some level of protection against some STD and HIV. Additional studies are currently underway to assess the effectiveness of female condoms against HIV and other STD as well as to develop additional methods of contraception for women.

**10. Isn't abstinence the only foolproof way to prevent HIV infection?**

Refraining from intercourse with infected partners is the most effective HIV prevention strategy. This is an especially important message for young people. There is little disagreement that premature initiation of sexual activity carries health risks. We need to strive for a climate supportive of young people who are choosing to delay sexual activity.

Periodic abstinence, however, carries with it certain risks. A 1988 *National Survey of Family Growth* found abstinence to have a contraceptive failure rate of 26% when not practiced consistently. So, in abstinence—as in condom use—consistency is key.

**11. Why are you changing your position on the effectiveness of condoms used in conjunction with a spermicide?**

Scientific studies show that condoms are more effective than many people previously thought and that spermicides may be less effective than had been hoped. CDC recommendations actually are not changing significantly. We are reinforcing the recommendation to use condoms. We don't encourage the use of spermicides except as an adjunct to condoms and for those whose goal is contraception.

**12. Is the federal government advocating/condoning sexual intercourse outside of marriage?**

There are many sound public health reasons to abstain from sexual intercourse, such as preventing STD, including HIV, and unwanted pregnancy. However, the federal government does not determine what is or is not morally acceptable behavior. From a public health perspective, if a person chooses to have sexual intercourse, using condoms correctly every time during sex is the best way to prevent HIV infection.

**13. Why are you releasing this information now? Aren't people already using condoms?**

We are releasing this information now because recently presented scientific data sheds new light on this important public health issue. We feel the public needs this information, and the *MMWR* is the most rapid means to disseminate it to health professionals and the public.

Most sexually active people are not using latex condoms every time they have sex. For example, in San Francisco, only 6% of heterosexual males with multiple sex partners reported always using condoms. In another study, only about 20% of sexually active American women reported that their male partners used condoms. And a national survey of heterosexual adults with multiple sex partners found only 17% used condoms all of the time (Catania et al., 1992).

One of the key determinants of condom use is the belief that they work. Therefore, it is important for sexually active individuals to get the message that latex condoms can provide effective protection from HIV if they are used correctly and consistently.

**14. Don't education programs about condoms result in increased sexual activity among adolescents?**

No. Several studies have shown that levels of sexual activity among young adults decreased or remained the same after sex education programs which included information about condoms. In a recent Swiss study of 16 to 19 year olds, an HIV prevention effort focusing on condom use did not increase the level of sexual activity or the number of sex partners of young people. However, condom use did increase among those already sexually active. A 1992 study reported in *Family Planning Perspectives* found that HIV education and sexuality education resulted in decreases in the number of sex partners and the frequency of intercourse. Having received education was also associated with more consistent condom use.

**15. In choosing a condom, is there any way to know which brand is best? Do some condoms have higher quality standards than others?**

All of the condoms marketed in the United States today meet federal quality assurance standards. The CDC recommends latex condoms for prevention of HIV and STD. Consumers should look for the word "latex" on the package. Color, shape and packaging are all issues of personal preference. All are effective.

**16. What are you going to do now that you have this information? Is the government going to start a condom promotion campaign? Are you going to release ads on condoms?**

The CDC is now planning the next stage of its HIV Public Information Program. It will include the implementation of a five-year prevention marketing program to prevent the sexual transmission of HIV among sexually active young Americans.

The CDC is faced with opposition regarding condoms from both sides of the issue. Some people want the CDC to promote only abstinence as a strategy to prevent HIV and not to discuss condoms at all. Others say the CDC is not talking enough about condoms.

The CDC's education programs are driven by science. As the nation's leading prevention agency, our mission is to prevent disease and protect the health of all Americans. For people who are sexually active, it is our duty to provide them with accurate, scientific information about the effectiveness of condoms against STD, including HIV, when condoms are used correctly and consistently. CDC-supported public health and education programs provide young Americans with information about the actions they can take to reduce their risk of acquiring HIV infection, including delaying and abstaining from sexual activity.

**17. Why are you promoting this information now?**

Two recent studies—especially the discordant couple studies—have provided the data to make a compelling new case for condom effectiveness.

**18. Why are you promoting condoms even though they're not foolproof?**

Because latex condoms substantially reduce the risk of HIV infection during vaginal, anal or oral sex. Similarly, we promote many other health behaviors that significantly reduce risk, but do not entirely eliminate it. For example, we promote wearing bicycle helmets, which are 85 percent effective at reducing injury or death, and wearing safety belts, which are 40 to 55 percent effective at reducing injury.

# References

Catania, J. A., et al. 1992. Prevalence of AIDS-related risk factors and condom use in the United States. *Science Magazine*, 13 November.

*Consumer Reports*. 1989. Can you rely on condoms? March.

DeVincenzi, I., and the European Study Group on Heterosexual Transmission of HIV. 1993. Heterosexual transmission of HIV in a European cohort of couples. Ninth International Conference on AIDS, 9 June, Berlin. (Abstract WSC02-1.)

Dubois-Arber, F., A. Jeannin and P. Zeugin. 1992. Evaluation of AIDS prevention in Switzerland: Behavioral change in the general population. Paper presented at the Eighth International Conference on AIDS, 19-24 July, Amsterdam. (Abstract PoD5140.)

Hausser, D., and P. A. Michaud. 1992. Condom promotion does not increase sexual intercourse among adolescents. Paper presented at the Eighth International Conference on AIDS, 19-24 July, Amsterdam. (Abstract TuD0575.)

Ku, L. C., F. L. Sonenstein and J. H. Pleck. 1992. The association of AIDS education and sex education with sexual behavior and condom use among teenage men. *Family Planning Perspectives* 24 (3): 100-106.

Richters, J., B. Donovan, J. Gerofi and L. Watson. 1988. Low condom breakage rate in commercial sex [letter]. *Lancet* 2 (8626/8627): 1487-1488.

Roper, W. L., H. B. Peterson and J. W. Curran. 1993. Commentary: Condoms and HIV/STD prevention—clarifying the message. *American Journal of Public Health* 83 (4): 501-502.

Saracco, A., M. Musicco, A. Nocolos et al. 1993. Man-to-woman sexual transmission of HIV: Longitudinal study of 343 steady partners of infected men. *Journal of Acquired Immune Deficiency Syndromes* 6 (5): 497-502.

Trussell, J., R. A. Hatcher, W. Cates, F. H. Stewart and K. Kost. Contraceptive failure in the United States: An update. *Studies in Family Planning* 21:51-54.

Voeller, B., A. H. Coulson, G. S. Bernstein et al. 1989. Mineral oil lubricants cause rapid deterioration of latex condoms. *Contraception* 39 (1): 95-102.